# HEALTH PROMOTION & WELLBEING IN PEOPLE WITH MENTAL HEALTH PROBLEMS

EDITED BY

# TIM BRADSHAW    HILARY MAIRS

# HEALTH PROMOTION &
# WELLBEING
## IN PEOPLE WITH
## MENTAL HEALTH PROBLEMS

## $SAGE

Los Angeles | London | New Delhi
Singapore | Washington DC | Melbourne

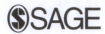

Los Angeles | London | New Delhi
Singapore | Washington DC | Melbourne

SAGE Publications Ltd
1 Oliver's Yard
55 City Road
London EC1Y 1SP

SAGE Publications Inc.
2455 Teller Road
Thousand Oaks, California 91320

SAGE Publications India Pvt Ltd
B 1/I 1 Mohan Cooperative Industrial Area
Mathura RoadA
New Delhi 110 044

SAGE Publications Asia-Pacific Pte Ltd
3 Church Street
#10-04 Samsung Hub
Singapore 049483

Editor: Becky Taylor
Assistant editor: Charlène Burin
Production editor: Katie Forsythe
Proofreader: Mary Dalton
Indexer: Adam Pozner
Marketing manager: Tamara Navaratnam
Cover design: Wendy Scott
Typeset by: C&M Digitals (P) Ltd, Chennai, India
Printed by CPI Group (UK) Ltd,
Croydon, CR0 4YY

**Library of Congress Control Number: 2016952632**

**British Library Cataloguing in Publication data**

A catalogue record for this book is available from
the British Library

ISBN 978-1-4739-5195-2
ISBN 978-1-4739-5196-9 (pbk)

At SAGE we take sustainability seriously. Most of our products are printed in the UK using FSC papers and boards.
When we print overseas we ensure sustainable papers are used as measured by the PREPS grading system.
We undertake an annual audit to monitor our sustainability.

In memory of Brian ...

# CONTENTS

# LIST OF FIGURES AND TABLES

## FIGURES

## TABLES

# PUBLISHER'S ACKNOWLEDGEMENTS

The Publishers would also like to thank the following lecturers for their invaluable feedback on the proposal and draft chapters:

Angelina Chadwick, University of Salford, UK

Sonya Chelvanayagam, Bournemouth University, UK

Keith Ford, Northumbria University, UK

Rebecca Rylance, Liverpool John Moores University, UK

The authors and publishers are grateful to the following for their kind permission to reproduce material:

Figure 1.1: The copyright and all other intellectual property rights in the material to be reproduced are owned by, or licensed to, the Commission for Equality and Human Rights, known as the Equality and Human Rights Commission ('the EHRC') (full document *Equal Treatment: Closing the Gap. A Formal Investigation into Physical Health Inequalities Experienced by People with Learning Disabilities and/or Mental Health Problems* available at: http://disability-studies.leeds.ac.uk/files/library/DRC-Health-FI-main.pdf).

Table 2.1: Reproduced from Crawford, M.J., Jayakumar, S., Lemmey, S.J. et al. (2014) 'Assessment and treatment of physical health problems among people with schizophrenia: national cross-sectional study', *British Journal of Psychiatry*, 205: 473–7. Available at: http://bjp.rcpsych.org/content/bjprcpsych/205/6/473.full.pdf with permission from *British Journal of Psychiatry*.

Table 3.1: Reproduced from Chest pain, in *The BMJ*, Christopher Bass, Richard Mayo, 325, 2002, with permission from BMJ Publishing Group Ltd.

Figure 8.1: Reproduced from McManus, S., Meltzer, H. and Campion, J. (2010) *Cigarette Smoking and Mental Health in England: Data from the Adult Psychiatric Morbidity Survey 2007*. London: National Centre for Social Research. Available at: www.natcen.ac.uk/media/21994/smoking-mental-health.pdf (accessed 25 August 2016), with permission of the National Centre for Smoking Cessation and Training (NCSCT).

Table 8.1: Reproduced from Shahab, L. (2013) *Quick Wins: The Short-Term Benefits of Stopping Smoking: Full Report, National Centre for Smoking Cessation and Training (NCSCT)*. Available at: www.ncsct.co.uk/usr/pub/Quick%20_wins_full_report.pdf (accessed 25 August 2016), with permission of the National Centre for Smoking Cessation and Training (NCSCT).

Table 9.1: Reprinted with permission from WHO (2016b) *Obesity and Overweight: Fact Sheet*. Updated June 2016. Available at: www.who.int/mediacentre/factsheets/fs311/en/ (accessed 25 August 2016).

# ABOUT THE EDITORS AND AUTHORS

## THE EDITORS

**Tim Bradshaw** is a Reader in the division of Nursing, Midwifery and Social Work at Manchester University. He is also Programme Director of the Advanced Practice Interventions in Mental Health course and a Senior Fellow of the Higher Education Academy. Tim originally qualified as an adult nurse in 1986 before going into mental health nursing a year later. Tim has spent most of his career working with people who experience psychosis and has a particular interest in improving their physical health and wellbeing. Since completing his PhD in 2007, in which he evaluated a health education intervention for people with mental health problems, he has been involved in research about weight management and smoking cessation. He has also developed a short course about physical health and wellbeing for mental health professionals and has published numerous articles on this subject.

**Hilary Mairs** is a Reader and the Director of Postgraduate Education in the School of Health Sciences at Manchester University. She worked in a range of NHS mental health settings providing both occupational and cognitive behavioural therapies, before beginning her academic career at Manchester University in 2002. Her teaching and scholarly interests focus on developing and delivering education and training for mental health professionals working in a range of settings. She is also a chartered psychologist, a Senior Fellow of the Higher Education Academy and the Chair of the Board of Trustees for Connect Support, a Manchester-based charity supporting carers of people with mental health problems.

## THE AUTHORS

**Rebekah Carney** is a researcher at Manchester University, working on her PhD in Medicine. Rebekah has a BSc in Psychology and an MSc in Clinical and Cognitive Neuroimaging. Her PhD research is focused on improving the physical health of young people with emerging psychological difficulties, particularly those at ultra-high risk for psychosis. Rebekah has a keen interest in behaviour change and health promotion to improve physical and mental health, and has published in both medical and nursing journals. She is also interested in behavioural risk factors, such as substance use in at-risk groups.

**Jackie Cleator** is an Adult Field Lecturer in the division of Nursing, Midwifery and Social Work at Manchester University and is the Academic Lead for Quality Assurance. Prior to joining the university in 2012, she worked for several years as a clinical researcher focusing on diabetes and obesity, and as an extended scope practitioner and operational manager of specialist obesity services. An interest in obesity-related eating behaviours developed from her clinical practice and led to her undertaking a PhD in night-time eating. She is a National Fellow of the Specialist Certification of Obesity Professional Education Programme (SCOPE) for the World Obesity Federation and contributes to the development and review of study modules. She is particularly committed to embedding knowledge and understanding of obesity in undergraduate curricula.

**Patricia Conaghan** is a Senior Lecturer in Adult Nursing in the division of Nursing, Midwifery and Social Work at Manchester University. Her clinical background is in Acute Medicine and Coronary Care, where she developed a specialist interest in resuscitation. She is a Fellow of the European Resuscitation Council and Chair of the Education Working Group and works with the Resuscitation Council (UK) as an Educator. She has previously held senior management posts in the NHS, with experience in Clinical Governance, Risk Management and General Management. Because of her experiences managing risk in the NHS, she is committed to improving patient safety through the education and training of staff.

**Joseph Firth** completed his undergraduate degree in Psychology at Sheffield University in 2012. He is now in the final year of his PhD in Medicine at Manchester University. His research focuses on developing and evaluating novel interventions to facilitate symptomatic and functional recovery in serious mental disorders. Specifically, the majority of his work has been on using physical exercise as an intervention for first-episode psychosis.

**Nigel Henderson** is a Senior Lecturer in the division of Nursing, Midwifery and Social Work at Manchester University. He qualified as an adult nurse in 1982, working in general and transplant surgery, eventually specialising in adult intensive care. In 1991, he entered nurse education and has since developed a specialist interest in the teaching and learning of the biosciences within nursing and allied health. He completed his PhD in 2015, in which he explored the area of textbook choice and how these texts supported learning within the biosciences. In addition to being a registered nurse, he is also a Principal Fellow of the Higher Education Academy and actively promotes the value of the biosciences within nurse education and clinical practice and how it underpins many aspects of nursing care assessment, planning, implementation and evaluation.

**David Shiers** is an Honorary Reader in Early Psychosis at Manchester University. Qualifying in Medicine in 1974, David settled happily into general practice in North Staffordshire. Things changed when his daughter developed schizophrenia in the late 1990s. From initial complaints about care offered to his daughter for schizophrenia, David became involved in radical Early Intervention in Psychosis reform to help other families avoid the experiences that his family had in this. David eventually made a major career change to jointly lead with Professor Jo Smith England's Early Intervention in Psychosis Development Programme (Smith and Shiers, 2014). As a former GP, David continues to challenge why people like his daughter should accept poor physical health, participating in relevant NICE guideline and quality standards, as clinical advisor to National Audits of Schizophrenia (2011–15), and co-leading Healthy Active Lives (Shiers and Curtis, 2014; International Physical Health in Youth (iphYs) Working Group, 2013), an international consensus on intervening early to protect people's bodies as well as minds.

**Jacquie White** has been a registered mental health nurse since 1986. She studied the role of the mental health nurse in medication management on the acute unit for her first degree and conducted a programme of research into physical health checks in secondary mental health services for her PhD. Developing practice that has an impact on the health of people with serious mental illness remains the focus of her teaching, research and scholarship activity. Jacquie has worked at the Faculty of Health and Social Care at Hull University since 2002. She was promoted to Senior Lecturer in 2011 and is now the Associate Dean Learning Teaching and Quality.

**Ian Wilson** is a mental health nurse. He is also a Clinical Teaching Fellow at the division of Nursing, Midwifery and Social Work at Manchester University and dual diagnosis trainer/clinical nurse in the Manchester Dual Diagnosis Liaison Service, Manchester Mental Health and Social Care Trust. He has a particular interest in the application of evidence-based interventions for people with complex mental health needs and substance misuse problems, working with carers of 'dually diagnosed' service users and the delivery of cognitive behavioural family therapy. Additionally, he attempts to address the training needs of a wide range of workers who come into contact with clients with complex needs.

# PREFACE

This book has been written as a practical guide to help health practitioners develop the knowledge and skills required to address the significant health disparities that people with mental health problems face in relation to their physical health. It is unacceptable that people with mental health problems have poor physical health, in addition to distressing experiences and a reduced life expectancy of up to 20 years. The early chapters of the book explore these disparities in further detail and examine the reasons for this. Chapters 5 and 6 detail the need to intervene in early stages to minimise the risks of long-term physical ill health. Chapters 7 to 9 offer a series of evidence-based strategies to address a number of lifestyle factors, including diet, exercise and smoking. In Chapter 10, we offer an evidence-based tool to enhance the detection of physical health problems so that optimal treatments can be put in place. The final two chapters offer two psychological approaches to enhance activity levels and instil the motivation to participate in the evidence-based interventions that we have outlined.

# MENTAL AND PHYSICAL HEALTH IN CONTEXT

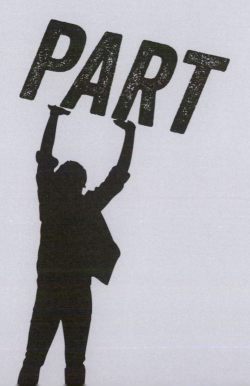

PART

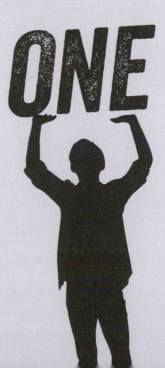

ONE

# ONE

## CONCEPTS OF HEALTH AND CURRENT HEALTH POLICY

### TIM BRADSHAW

### CHAPTER LEARNING OUTCOMES

After reading this chapter, you will be able to:

- Understand the language and terminology of public health.
- Access public health data in order to examine the health needs of different communities.
- Explore modifiable and unmodifiable risk factors for poor physical health and wellbeing in people with mental health problems.
- Examine current UK health policy in relation to the physical health of people with mental health problems.

## MULTIPLE CHOICE QUESTIONS

We have included 10 multiple choice questions at the beginning of this chapter for readers wishing to test their knowledge of its contents. We have included the answers at the end of the chapter, but advise you not to check these until you have answered them before and after reading the chapter so that you can determine how much your knowledge has increased.

1. Patterns of health, illness and mortality are studied through which of the following sciences:

   a) Sociology
   b) Epidemiology
   c) Criminology
   d) Biology

*(Continued)*

*(Continued)*

2. The term 'morbidity' refers to which of the following:

   a) The number of new cases of an illness in a given population over a defined period of time.
   b) The number of overall cases of an illness in a given population at a specific point in time.
   c) The number of deaths in a given population over a given period of time.
   d) Patterns of illness in a given population.

3. If there are 400 people with type 2 diabetes in a community of 10,000 what is the prevalence of this condition?

   a) 10%
   b) 4%
   c) 0.4%
   d) 40%

4. According to the World Health Organization (WHO, 2015), which of the following countries has the highest life expectancy in the world:

   a) England
   b) Germany
   c) Japan
   d) China

5. Brown et al. (2010) found that the death rate from endocrine disease in people with schizophrenia was more than four times higher than in the general population. Which of the following might represent the standardised mortality ratio (SMR) for the condition:

   a) 443
   b) 46
   c) 800
   d) 104

6. Which of the following is a modifiable risk factor for poor physical health:

   a) Age
   b) Gender
   c) Prescription of an atypical antipsychotic medication
   d) Family history

7. According to the General Medical Services contract 2004, how often should people with serious mental illness be offered a physical health check by their GP?

   a) Annually
   b) Monthly
   c) Bi-annually
   d) Every 5 years

8. Which of the following is recommended for use by mental health nurses in NHS England's (2016a) report, *Improving the Physical Health of People with Serious Mental Illness: A Practical Toolkit*:

   a) The Health Improvement Profile (HIP) for Serious Mental Illness assessment.
   b) The Rethink Physical Health Check.

c) The Primary Care Guidance on Smoking and Mental Disorders.
d) The Lester Positive Cardiometabolic Health Resource.

9. According to Brown et al. (2010), in a cohort of people with schizophrenia, what percentage of excess mortality was attributable to death from unnatural causes such as suicides and accidents?

a) 66%
b) 45%
c) 26%
d) 17%

10. Which report published by Health Education England in 2015 has recommended a change in pre-registration nurse education to enhance shared learning between students from adult and mental health fields in the first two years of their course?

a) *Shape of Caring* review
b) *Project 2020*
c) *Parity of Esteem* review
d) *Health of the Nation*

# INTRODUCTION

People with mental health problems commonly experience co-morbid physical health conditions such as cardiovascular diseases (CVD), respiratory diseases and metabolic disorders. Naylor et al. (2012) have estimated that 20% of the population in England has a mental health problem (about 10.2 million people) and that 46% of this group also have a physical health condition (about 4.6 million people). These latter 4.6 million people are two to four times more likely to die prematurely from the 'natural' causes identified above (ibid.). While this book focuses on this population, it is worth noting that there is also clear evidence that having a long-term physical health problem – such as cardiovascular disease, diabetes, chronic obstructive pulmonary disease (COPD) or chronic musculoskeletal disorders – increases the risk of then having a number of co-morbid mental health problems, including anxiety and depression (ibid.). For example, people with diabetes are two to three times more likely to experience depression than other members of the general population (Simon et al., 2007; Vamos et al., 2009), and panic disorder is up to ten times more prevalent in people living with COPD (Livermore et al., 2010). Clearly the relationship between mental health and physical health conditions is a two-way process (Naylor et al., 2012). We have already used terms that feature in the epidemiology literature (e.g. co-morbid and prevalent) and, in this chapter, we introduce these and other key concepts of epidemiology (patterns of health, illness and mortality) and public health (the art and science of promoting health, preventing disease and prolonging life) (Nash, 2014) in order to set the scene for this book and establish the associations between the onset of mental health problems, poor physical health and premature mortality.

## INCIDENCE

'Incidence' is the term used to describe the number of new cases of an illness in a given population over a defined period of time. For example, if 500 new cases of a specific illness are identified over the course of one year in a population of 100,000 people, the incidence of that illness is 0.5% (500/100,000 x 100).

The incidence of mental health problems varies across different diagnostic categories. Approximately 1 in 4 people will experience a common mental health problem such as anxiety and depression each year but the incidence of serious mental illness such as psychosis is much lower (Kirkbride et al., 2012). Studies show that the incidence of many common medical problems, including diabetes (Hsu et al., 2011), stroke (Tsai et al., 2012) and cardiovascular disease (Callaghan et al., 2009), are all higher in people with mental health problems than in other members of the general population.

## COMORBIDITY

'Morbidity' is the term used to describe patterns of illness in a specified population or specific setting. When more than one illness is present in the population under scrutiny, this is referred to as 'comorbidity'. For example, in excess of 20% of people over 55 years of age with chronic arthritis of the knee are reported to have co-morbid depression (Sale et al., 2008). At the same time, research consistently demonstrates that people living with mental health problems (a diagnosis of schizophrenia or

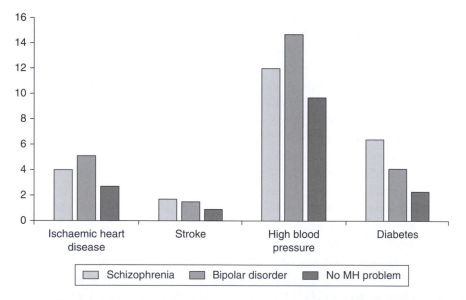

**Figure 1.1   Prevalence of physical health problems amongst people with schizophrenia or bipolar disorder**

*Source*: Data taken from Disability Rights Commission (2006), reproduced with kind permission of the Commission for Equality and Human Rights

bipolar disorder) are more likely to develop co-morbid physical health problems such as ischaemic heart disease, stroke, high blood pressure and diabetes than people without mental health problems (Figure 1.1). In addition, they are significantly more likely to develop these physical health problems before the age of 55 and have poorer 5-year survival rates once diagnosed (Disability Rights Commission, 2006).

## PREVALENCE

The term 'prevalence' refers to the number of overall cases of an illness in a given population at a specific point in time. If we return to our community of 100,000 people again and find that there are 2900 known cases of a specific illness, then its prevalence is 2.9% (2900/100,000 x 100). Calculating the incidence and prevalence of different physical health problems in a given population is important because it may help us to spot associations and identify possible causal factors for these conditions.

As shown in Figure 1.1, the prevalence of several common medical conditions is higher in people with mental health problems at a younger age than in others without mental health problems.

## LIFE EXPECTANCY

Life expectancy, the number of years a person can expect to live from birth until death has steadily improved since the Second World War, but is still subject to geographical variation. For example, the longest and shortest life expectancy across the world is currently estimated at 83.7 years in Japan and 50.1 years in Sierra Leone (WHO, 2015). In the UK, life expectancy in men and women is 79.1 and 82.9 years, respectively (Office of National Statistics, 2016). Brown et al. (2010) found that the average age of death in a sample of 370 people with schizophrenia living in the south of England was 57.3 years in men and 65.5 years in women, showing that life expectancy was reduced by 21 years and 17 years, respectively. Furthermore, a recently published meta-review (a review of systematic reviews) found that life expectancy is reduced by 7–11 years for depression, 9–24 years for substance misuse, 13–22 years for personality disorder, 10–20 years for schizophrenia and 9–20 years for bipolar disorder (Chesney et al., 2014). To put this into perspective, it means that life expectancy in people with schizophrenia in England is worse than that of the general population of most countries in the world, with the exception of a small number of countries in Sub-Saharan Africa (WHO, 2015).

## MORTALITY RATE

The 'mortality rate' is the number of deaths in a given population over a given period of time. Mortality rates help to determine the biggest causes of death and allow the examination of these causes in different subgroups of the population by looking at such factors as age, gender, ethnicity, social class, etc. Mortality rates resulting from unnatural causes of death such as suicide have been shown to be over 10 times higher in people with mental health problems. However, this still only accounts for 17% of excess mortality, with 82% being attributable to deaths resulting from 'natural' causes such as cardiovascular disease (Brown et al., 2010).

# STANDARDISED MORTALITY RATIO (SMR)

The 'standardised mortality ratio' represents the ratio between the expected number of deaths from a particular health problem in a given population and the actual number observed. The average standardised mortality ratio is normally expressed as either a 1 or 100, and any number larger than this figure would suggest a higher than expected death rate for that condition. Standardised mortality ratios are useful in a number of ways. They can help:

- Establish potential causal links between lifestyle behaviours and illnesses, for example smoking and death from lung cancer (Doll et al., 2004).
- Compare rates of death from different conditions in different communities or parts of the country.
- Establish rates of death in subgroups of the community such as people with mental health problems compared to others.

The standardised mortality ratio for most common physical health problems in people with mental health problems has been shown to be consistently two to three times higher compared to others in the general population (Brown et al., 2010).

## ACTIVITY 1.1   ACCESSING DATA ON THE HEALTH OF DIFFERENT COMMUNITIES IN ENGLAND

The standardised mortality ratio for most common medical conditions in different electoral wards across England can be accessed and compared with the country's averages by visiting Public Health England's website and following the instructions below:

- Click www.localhealth.org.uk/#l=en;v=map4 you should then see the 'Welcome to Local Health' page.
- From the menu above the heading, 'Welcome to Local Health', select 'FIND MY AREA'.
- Click 'Choose an area'.
- Put your area's name into the search box, e.g. 'Cheetham'.
- Click the area's name when it appears in the box below.
- Click 'Information on selection'.
- Click 'Reports'.

- Click 'Profile'.
- A table should appear on the right-hand side that compares the data for your area with that of the average for England, including if you scroll down all key standardised mortality ratios.

Using this website, you can examine how healthy the area in which you live and work is compared to the rest of the country. If your area has high standardised mortality ratios for any conditions, reflect on what the reasons for this might be.

# FACTORS AFFECTING PHYSICAL AND MENTAL HEALTH

Data from Public Health England's website confirms that significant differences in life expectancy exist between communities that are often in close proximity to one another geographically.

## ACTIVITY 1.2    COMPARING THE HEALTH PROFILE OF DIFFERENT COMMUNITIES

Using the Public Health England website as described in Activity 1.1, compare the health of the populations of Cheetham with that of West Didsbury – these are both electoral wards of Manchester and geographically only five miles apart:

What can you conclude about the health of the two communities?

Interestingly, such health inequalities may equally apply to mental health as they do to physical health. For example, Kirkbride et al. (2007) found that the incidence of schizophrenia varied significantly across wards in South-East London, according to variations in neighbourhood-level risk factors such as ethnic density and social capital.

Attempting to understand factors that affect health and life expectancy in different populations may help us to understand the health inequalities that exist for people with mental health problems. Broadly speaking, risk factors for poor physical and mental health can be classified as being either modifiable or unmodifiable. Modifiable risk factors are those that we have some control over such as diet and exercise, whilst non-modifiable risk factors are not within our control and include things such as family history and age.

Whilst there is little evidence that people with mental health problems have more unmodifiable risk factors for poor physical health than others in the general population, there is strong evidence that they are disproportionately exposed to a greater number of modifiable risk factors. Throughout this book, we will discuss ways in which practitioners can begin to reduce health inequalities in people with mental health problems by helping them to develop healthier and happier lifestyles and protecting them from the harmful effects of some of the medications used to treat their mental health problems.

## GOVERNMENT POLICY RELATED TO THE PHYSICAL HEALTH AND WELLBEING OF PEOPLE WITH MENTAL HEALTH PROBLEMS

For the past decade, successive reports and government policies have recognised the unacceptable health inequalities experienced by people with mental health problems and started to make recommendations for how these might be addressed. In 2004, the General Medical Services Contract (Roland, 2004) incentivised GPs via the Quality Outcomes Framework (NHS digital, 2016) to develop Serious Mental Illness case registers and to conduct annual physical health checks with all those on their register. The National Institute for Health and Care Excellence (NICE, 2009: clinical guideline (CG)82) provided best practice recommendations for the assessment and monitoring of physical health in adults with schizophrenia, including recommendations regarding improving the interface between primary and secondary care services. The updated guidelines by NICE (2014a: CG178) also contain a whole chapter devoted to outlining interventions to promote physical health in adults with schizophrenia or psychosis.

More recent government policy has reasserted a commitment to reducing health inequalities and has recognised the importance of placing equal value on the prevention and treatment of both mental and physical health problems, calling for 'parity of esteem' between the two (Department of Health, 2014; Parliamentary Office of Science and Technology, 2015). This has been recognised in Health Education England's (2015) recent report *The Shape of Caring*, which makes recommendations for a change in the model of pre-registration nurse education to enhance shared learning between students from adult and mental health fields in the first two years of their training.

The most recent joint publication from the Department of Health and Public Health England (NHS England, 2016a), released in May 2016, advises mental health nurses about how they can improve the physical health of service users. This report again emphasises the importance of a holistic approach to the care of mental and physical health due to the complex relationship between the two. A practical toolkit has also been released to complement the report (NHS England, 2016b). This document focuses on lessons learned regarding the implementation of the Lester Positive Cardiometabolic Health Resource (see Chapter 6 for further details) in four NHS Trusts that acted as pilot sites between 2014 and 2016.

# CONCLUSION

In this chapter, we have examined some key concepts and terminology regarding epidemiology and public health. We provided instructions for how to use Public Health England's website to access epidemiological data about the health and longevity of different communities. On each of the key metrics discussed, we demonstrated that significant health inequalities exist in people with mental health problems compared with others in the general population. We then considered modifiable and unmodifiable risk factors for poor physical health, concluding that the health of people with mental health problems is disproportionately affected by modifiable risk factors that may be responsive to the interventions outlined in the chapters of this book. Finally, we provided a brief review of recent health policy and legislation which has been published in an attempt to address these inequalities for people with mental health problems.

# USEFUL RESOURCES

National Institute for Health and Care Excellence (NICE) (2014a) *Psychosis and Schizophrenia in Adults: Treatment and Management*. Available at: http://www.nice.org.uk/Guidance/CG178 (accessed 4 August 2016).

The most recently published NICE guidelines provide details of a range of evidence-based approaches for improving the mental and physical health of people experiencing psychosis and schizophrenia.

NHS England (2016) *Improving the Physical Health of People with Mental Health Problems: Actions for Mental Health Nurses*. Available at: www.gov.uk/government/uploads/system/uploads/attachment_data/file/532253/JRA_Physical_Health_revised.pdf (accessed 4 August 2016).

This report describes eight aspects of physical health where a mental health nurse can take action to improve the health of service users.

# ANSWERS TO MULTIPLE CHOICE QUESTIONS

1(b), 2(d), 3(b), 4(c), 5(a), 6(c), 7(a), 8(d), 9(d), 10(a)

# TWO

## PHYSICAL HEALTH IN PEOPLE WITH MENTAL HEALTH PROBLEMS

### TIM BRADSHAW

### CHAPTER LEARNING OUTCOMES

After reading this chapter, you will be able to:

- Consider the main reasons for poor physical health in people with mental health problems.
- Highlight the unacceptable 'scandal of premature mortality' in this client group.
- Describe a range of evidence-based strategies that can be used to promote better physical health and wellbeing.

### MULTIPLE CHOICE QUESTIONS

We have included 10 multiple choice questions at the beginning of this chapter for readers wishing to test their knowledge of its contents. We have included the answers at the end of the chapter, but advise you not to check these until you have answered them before and after reading the chapter so that you can determine how much your knowledge has increased.

1. Which of the following is *not* an explanation for the poor physical health of people with mental health problems:

   a) Adverse health behaviours such as smoking.
   b) Side effects of psychiatric medication.
   c) Lack of integration of health care services.
   d) Apathy and disinterest in physical health by service users.

2. People with serious mental illness may have problems with self-care due to:

   a) Their carers doing too much for them.
   b) Negative symptoms associated with the illness.
   c) Lack of knowledge about household management.
   d) Services not doing enough for them.

3. In people with serious mental illness, cancer is:

   a) Diagnosed earlier than in others.
   b) Twice as prevalent as in the general population.
   c) Diagnosed later and less aggressively managed.
   d) Uncommon.

4. Which types of physical health problems have a higher prevalence in people with mental health problems?

   a) Cardiovascular disease.
   b) Diabetes.
   c) Respiratory diseases.
   d) All of the above.

5. People with mental health problems:

   a) Eat poorer diets than others in the general population.
   b) Have lower levels of physical activity than others in the general population.
   c) Smoke more than others in the general population.
   d) All of the above.

6. What did Foley and Morley (2011) find the average weight gain for those taking the atypical antipsychotic medication olanzapine to be in the first 6–8 weeks of treatment in drug naive patients:

   a) 2–4kg
   b) 16–20kg
   c) 8–10kg
   d) 5–6kg

7. According to Firth et al. (2015), in people with mental health problems, 90 minutes of moderate-to-vigorous exercise per week has been shown to:

   a) Have no effect on functioning or psychiatric symptoms.
   b) Significantly reduce psychiatric symptoms but have no effect on functioning.
   c) Significantly improve functioning but have no effect on psychiatric symptoms.
   d) Significantly reduce psychiatric symptoms and improve functioning.

8. According to the International Diabetes Federation (2006), which of the following have been shown to contribute to a diagnosis of metabolic syndrome:

   a) Increased body mass index (BMI) and elevated blood pressure (BP).
   b) Abdominal (visceral) obesity and elevated blood pressure.
   c) Weight loss and elevated fasting plasma glucose (blood sugar).
   d) Elevated fasting plasma glucose (blood sugar) and low blood pressure.

9. Which of the following most accurately describes primary prevention of ill health:

   a) Prescribing Metformin to control antipsychotic-related weight gain.
   b) Providing information about health and wellbeing to help people make healthy lifestyle choices.
   c) Early intervention to manage modifiable risk factors for poor health such as high blood pressure before it has a detrimental effect.
   d) Identification and management of established health problems such as diabetes, hypertension and coronary heart disease (CHD).

*(Continued)*

*(Continued)*

10. Which interventions has research shown to be effective in improving health and wellbeing in people with mental health problems?

    a) Smoking cessation.
    b) Weight management.
    c) Health screening.
    d) All of the above.


# INTRODUCTION

As noted in the previous chapter, people with mental health problems commonly experience the co-morbid physical health conditions that we have described in Chapter 1 (cardiovascular diseases, respiratory diseases and metabolic disorders such as diabetes) and are two to four times more likely to die prematurely from these so-called 'natural' causes. In this chapter, we explore the reasons for these health inequalities in further detail and introduce a range of evidence-based strategies to promote the health and wellbeing of people living with mental health problems.


# WHY DO PEOPLE WITH MENTAL HEALTH PROBLEMS HAVE POORER PHYSICAL HEALTH?

The mechanisms underlying the relationship between mental health problems and physical health conditions are complex and multifaceted. It is likely that a combination of behavioural, psychological, biological and environmental factors may all be involved. We think that for most people with mental health problems, poor physical health is likely to result from an interaction of the following four factors:

1. The consequences of developing a mental health problem.
2. The side effects of medication.
3. Adverse health behaviours and poorer self-care.
4. The lack of integrated services to respond effectively to both physical and mental health needs of this population.


## *CONSEQUENCES OF DEVELOPING A MENTAL HEALTH PROBLEM*

For some people, the consequences of developing a mental health problem can be as distressing and disabling as the mental health problem itself. Consequences may include loss of self-confidence, self-consciousness and low motivation and energy levels. Consider, for example, young people with first-episode psychosis who often withdraw from social support networks because of a fear of how others will respond to them, thus isolating themselves and reducing their opportunities for meaningful daytime activity, including exercise. Others might have fears that they may no longer be able to achieve their goals and aspirations in life, which may lead them to withdraw from activities that are enjoyable and/or promote a sense of mastery (Mairs, 2017).

## SIDE EFFECTS OF MEDICATION

A significant part of the explanation for elevated rates of physical health problems is the side effects of some of the antidepressant and antipsychotic medications prescribed for mental health problems that can be detrimental to physical health. For example, Hamer et al. (2011) found an association between the prescription of tricyclic antidepressants (a traditional treatment for depression, now used much less often) and cardiovascular diseases in a large Scottish study. Others, such as Andrews et al. (2012), have concluded that this group of medicines actually do more harm than good, given that they increase the risk of hyponatremia (low sodium in blood plasma), bleeding and stroke and do not always alleviate the low mood for which they are prescribed.

All antipsychotic medications, particularly the newer drugs collectively known as 'atypical antipsychotics', have the potential to cause weight gain (Kahn et al., 2008). A systematic review by Foley and Morley (2011) found that the average weight gain in the first 6–8 weeks of treatment with olanzapine was 5–6 kg in drug naive patients. Service users also began to show other unhealthy metabolic changes such as increases in insulin levels, insulin resistance, and glucose, cholesterol, triglyceride and C peptide levels. These side effects of atypical antipsychotics contribute to the abnormally high prevalence of metabolic syndrome observed in people with mental health problems (Mitchell et al., 2013b). Metabolic syndrome is associated with an increased risk of cardiovascular disease and diabetes and diagnosed by the presence of three out of the five metabolic abnormalities, as listed below:

1. Abdominal (visceral) obesity.
2. Elevated blood pressure.
3. Elevated fasting plasma glucose (blood sugar).
4. High serum triglycerides (circulating fat).
5. Low high-density (HDL, good) cholesterol level.
   International Diabetes Federation (2006, p. 10)

Studies have shown that compared to the general population, people with serious mental health problems are approximately twice as likely to have metabolic syndrome (Galletly et al., 2012). Steps to protect young people from these harmful side effects are explored in detail in Chapter 6.

## ADVERSE HEALTH BEHAVIOURS AND POOR SELF-CARE

A further part of the explanation for elevated rates of physical health problems is that mental health problems are associated with unhealthy behaviours such as smoking, a sedentary lifestyle and poor diet. We consider each in turn.

Smoking is the single most preventable cause of premature death from cancer, cardiovascular disease and respiratory disease in the global population, with the WHO (2016c) estimating that it kills 6 million people a year. People with mental health problems smoke more cigarettes than the general population do. Smoking in the general population averages 19% in England (Niblett, 2015), but rates increase to 33% in people with common mental health problems (McManus et al., 2010) and up to 70% in people with psychosis (Jochelson and Majrowski, 2006). These significantly elevated rates of smoking accounted for 70% of the excess mortality from 'natural' causes observed in a UK cohort of people with schizophrenia (Brown et al., 2010), and approximately 50% of all deaths in hospitals in the USA for people with psychosis, depression and bipolar (Callaghan et al., 2014). Evidence-based approaches to helping people with mental health problems to stop smoking will be described in Chapter 8.

The relationship between adequate levels of physical activity and better health is well established. It has been estimated that up to 37% of coronary heart disease in the UK may be attributed to low levels of physical activity (McPherson et al., 2002), and taking regular exercise is related to a reduced incidence of cardiovascular diseases, obesity, type 2 diabetes, many types of cancer and osteoporosis (Thompson et al., 2003). In addition to the beneficial effects of exercise on physical health, it also has therapeutic effects for many of the psychological symptoms associated with mental health problems (Morgan et al., 2013). These benefits will be reviewed in detail in Chapter 7, alongside strategies for helping people with mental problems to exercise more.

Only one third of UK adults meet the recommended amounts of exercise and levels of physical activity are even lower in people with mental health problems (Chapter 7). People with a diagnosis of schizophrenia engage in significantly less exercise and more sedentary behaviour than those in matched control groups (Soundy et al., 2013). At the same time, those who do not engage in regular moderate-to-vigorous exercise have poorer cardiorespiratory health and are at an increased risk of developing diabetes (Vancampfort et al., 2013).

Eating a healthy diet with an adequate intake of fruit and vegetables (five portions a day), and which is high in fibre and low in fat and salt, reduces the risk of heart disease and cancer (Huxley and Neil, 2003). A recent survey of 10,000 adults in the UK found that, on an average day, 64% of them did not eat the recommended 5-a-day portions of fruit and vegetables. In young people between the ages of 16–24 years, this figure increased to 79%. A number of studies have found that people with a diagnosis of schizophrenia eat less fruit than do other members of the general population and, in addition, their diets are more likely to be high in fat and refined sugar and low in fibre (Dipasquale et al., 2013).

As well as the adverse health behaviours outlined above, poor mental health can reduce the motivation and energy needed for self-care and management. For example, people with psychosis commonly lose interest and motivation in a range of everyday tasks (so-called 'negative symptoms'), including those required to take regular exercise or follow a healthy diet. Ways of helping people with the effects of negative symptoms are described in Chapter 11, whilst strategies for enhancing motivation are outlined in Chapter 12.

## THE LACK OF INTEGRATED SERVICES TO RESPOND EFFECTIVELY TO BOTH PHYSICAL AND MENTAL HEALTH NEEDS OF PEOPLE WITH MENTAL HEALTH PROBLEMS

A number of sources concur that services are poor at both recognition of and intervention for physical health problems in people with mental health problems. For example, Crawford et al. (2014) retrospectively audited the primary and secondary care notes of 5091 adults with a diagnosis of serious mental illness. Table 2.1 shows that, for the most important health indicators with the exception of use of tobacco, alcohol and substances, only about 50% of individuals had assessments recorded in their notes in the previous 12 months, showing routine physical health screening to be inadequate. Indeed, the authors conclude that:

> assessment and treatment of common physical health problems in people with schizophrenia falls well below acceptable standards. Cooperation and communication between primary and secondary care services needs to improve if premature mortality in this group is to be reduced. (Ibid.: 473)

Table 2.1 **Percentage of individuals with serious mental illness with documented evidence of assessment of physical health-related problems**

| Physical health indicator | % assessed |
| --- | --- |
| Weight | 56.3 |
| Body Mass Index (BMI) | 51.1 |
| Blood pressure | 56.2 |
| Blood glucose | 49.6 |
| Blood lipids (total cholesterol and high-density lipoprotein) | 47.0 |
| Tobacco use | 87.3 |
| Alcohol use | 69.1 |
| Substance use | 84.7 |

*Source*: Data taken from Crawford et al. (2014), reproduced with kind permission of the *British Journal of Psychiatry*

Since 2004, General Practitioners (GPs) in England have been incentivised via the Quality Outcomes Framework (QOF) to perform an annual physical health check on people with severe mental illness (Roland, 2004). QOF is a voluntary process for GPs to participate in, where they receive annual financial rewards for managing long-term health problems. Despite the QOF targets, Smith et al. (2013a) found that people with a diagnosis of schizophrenia were less likely to have a primary care record of cardiovascular disease, and the authors conclude that this suggests an under-recognition and under-treatment of the condition.

In addition, Hippisley-Cox et al. (2007) found that people with coronary heart disease who had a diagnosis of schizophrenia or bipolar disorder were 15% less likely to be prescribed statins and 7% less likely to have a recent record of their cholesterol levels. Somewhat surprisingly, given that all the following factors can be adversely affected by antipsychotic medication, the QOF indicators have recently been changed and GPs are no longer required to measure cholesterol, glucose/HbA1 or BMI (Guthrie and Morales, 2014).

Further evidence of under-recognition and under-treatment of physical health problems as listed below:

- Women with any type of non-organic psychiatric disorder are significantly less likely to receive mammography screening to detect breast cancer, with the lowest rates being observed in women with more serious mental health problems (Mitchell et al., 2014).
- After a cardiac event, people with mental health problems are 14% less likely to have invasive coronary procedures such as revascularisation, angiography, angioplasty and bypass grafting, which contributes to an 11% increased mortality rate. People with a diagnosis of schizophrenia are 47% less likely to have these procedures (Mitchell and Lawrence, 2011).
- People with mental health problems with a diagnosis of cancer are more likely to have metastases at presentation, suggesting lower levels of screening and early detection, and they are less likely to receive surgery, radiotherapy or chemotherapy to treat their cancer once it has been detected (Kisely et al., 2013).

Collectively, these studies suggest that health screening in people with mental health problems is inadequate and that, even when health problems are detected, they are often treated less aggressively than they would be in people without a diagnosis of a mental health problem. These inadequate responses of health services may further compound health inequality and premature mortality.

---

⚙ **REFLECTION POINT 2.1**

Think about the service that you work in/have worked in most recently:

- Were you aware of any initiatives or policies targeted specifically at improving the physical health and wellbeing of service users with mental health problems?
- Do you know what the driving forces for these initiatives are?

The Schizophrenia Commission (2012) report on the 'forgotten illness' argued that this neglect of the physical health of people with the diagnosis could not be allowed to continue, whilst Thornicroft (2011: 441) describes this gap in life expectancy as 'the scandal of premature mortality' representing 'a cynical disregard for the lost lives' of people with mental health problems who are valued less than others in our society. We now move on to explore a range of evidence-based interventions to promote better physical health and wellbeing in people with mental health problems that may address this 'scandal of premature mortality' (ibid.).

---

### ⚙ REFLECTION POINT 2.2

1. Make a list of as many different interventions as you can think of that may help to improve the physical health and wellbeing of people with mental health problems.
2. Do you know which interventions evidence suggests might be effective?
3. In your experience, how many of these interventions are currently routinely offered to service users in practice?

---

# INTERVENTIONS TO IMPROVE HEALTH AND WELLBEING

The literature suggests that opportunities to intervene to promote physical health and wellbeing should be provided as early as possible. In Chapter 5, we present evidence demonstrating that the risk factors for poor cardiovascular health, such as a high prevalence of smoking, substance abuse and lower levels of physical activity, are evident in young people at high risk of psychosis even before they make the transition to the illness. Consequently, we argue that lifestyle interventions targeted at this high-risk group may have benefits for both their mental and physical health. For example, Amminger et al. (2010) found that dietary supplements of long-chain omega-3 fatty acids significantly reduced the transition to psychosis in a group of 81 individuals at ultra-high risk of psychosis. Also, a recent systematic review by Gurillo et al. (2015) found a possible causative link between smoking tobacco and psychosis, suggesting that if young people could be discouraged from smoking in the first place, fewer new cases of psychosis may occur. Although this is early stage research, these studies nevertheless suggest that interventions that focus on the promotion of healthy eating and discouraging smoking may have dual benefits in terms of both mental and physical health in young people at high risk of psychosis.

Evidence that post transition to first-episode psychosis more risk factors for poor health such as weight gain and other metabolic disturbances can rapidly emerge due to the side effects of antipsychotic medication is presented in Chapter 6. We propose that the antecedents to future poor cardiometabolic health are entirely predictable in people with psychosis, and intervention at first episode may prevent the development of these problems.

Interventions such as weight management, promoting physical activity, smoking cessation and managing substance misuse may also be useful in those with more established mental health problems (Gates et al., 2015). A meta-analysis of 17 studies has confirmed that participation in non-pharmacological interventions (including cognitive behavioural therapy and nutritional approaches) results in a significant average weight loss of 3.12 kg in a large sample of overweight people (Caemmerer et al., 2012). A systematic review by Praharaj et al. (2011) showed that, for individuals who are not able to participate in non-pharmacological interventions, an antidiabetic drug called Metformin resulted in a 5.02 kg weight loss compared with a placebo at 12 weeks. In addition to its beneficial effects on weight loss, Bailey et al. (2012) argue that Metformin's efficacy and safety as a treatment for pre-diabetes have been proven for more than 60 years and that it should be considered for people with serious mental ill health if lifestyle modification has failed to control glucose impairment.

Approximately 50% of people with serious mental ill health who smoke would like to try to give up (Doherty, 2006), and evidence suggests that the smoking cessation interventions that work in the general population are equally effective with this client group without any worsening of mental health where this is stable (Banham and Gilbody, 2010). In Chapter 8, we describe in detail a bespoke intervention that was developed and tested in the first randomised controlled trial of smoking cessation in people with mental health problems to be conducted in the UK (Gilbody et al., 2015).

Findings of a recent meta-analysis by Firth et al. (2015) demonstrate that exercise can improve physical fitness and other cardiometabolic risk factors. Moderate-to-vigorous exercise of 90 minutes per week also significantly reduces psychiatric symptoms and improves functioning, having dual benefits for both physical and mental health. The benefits of exercise are reviewed in detail in Chapter 7.

---

### 👥 CASE STUDY 2.1

Susan was 22 years old when she was first diagnosed with bipolar disorder two years ago and had been prescribed Lithium carbonate and olanzapine. Since becoming ill, Susan rarely left her home, she had lost her self-confidence and gained 20 kg in weight. Her support time recovery (STR) worker encouraged Susan to go to the local authority gym with her and, although Susan was initially anxious about this, she agreed to go twice a week. After 12 weeks, Susan had lost 7 kg in weight, felt less drowsy and more self-confident and started to go to the gym most days on her own. In fact, she had even paid a subscription to a more up-market private gym.

---

In addition to the lifestyle interventions such as the ones described above, there is also a need for services to improve health screening in order to detect and manage emerging health problems at an early stage (Crawford et al., 2014). In Chapter 10, we introduce the serious mental illness Health Improvement Profile (HIP; see White et al., 2009), an evidence-based tool designed to help health care professionals assess physical health in people with serious mental illness and direct them towards appropriate evidence-based interventions. Widescale adoption of the HIP in routine clinical practice could go a long way towards helping services to address the poor physical health of this group.

## KEY MESSAGE 2.1

Research shows us that effective interventions can be made by health care professionals to improve the physical health of people with mental health problems. Interventions that have been evaluated include:

- Ones early in the illness that aim to stop problems like weight gain occurring (primary).
- Ones that help managing emerging risk factors for poor physical health such as weight gain and smoking (secondary).
- Health monitoring and screening to detect and initiate prompt management of emerging physical health problems such as diabetes (tertiary).

## CONCLUSION

In this chapter, we have explored the reasons for the poor physical health of people with mental health problems that include a combination of behavioural, psychological, biological and environmental factors. These factors combine to result in a pattern of unacceptable health inequality and premature death currently observed in this client group and which has been described as a violation of the 'right to health' as set out in Article 12 of International Covenant on Economic, Social and Cultural Rights (Thornicroft, 2011). We have also briefly described a range of interventions that have an emerging evidence base for their efficacy in improving the physical health and wellbeing of people with mental health problems, including smoking cessation, promoting exercise, weight management and health screening. Throughout the chapters that follow, each of these interventions will be explored in more detail and their implementation in practice described.

## USEFUL RESOURCES

Lester UK Adaptation (2015) *Positive Cardiometabolic Health Resource: An Intervention Framework for People Experiencing Psychosis and Schizophrenia*. Available at: www. rcgp.org.uk/clinical-and-research/clinical-resources/~/media/Files/CIRC/Mental%20 Health%20-%202014/10%20Lester%20Tool%20June%202014%20update%20 FINAL%20PDF.ashx (accessed 3 October 2016).

This user-friendly resource provides a visual illustration for mental health practitioners of the main aspects of cardiometabolic health, which should be monitored in people with serious mental illness, especially if they are prescribed antipsychotic medication. It highlights what constitutes abnormal assessment results and interventions that should be considered to promote positive cardiometabolic health.

Royal College of Psychiatrists website: *Improving Physical and Mental Health*. Available at: www.rcpsych.ac.uk/mentalhealthinfo/improvingphysicalandmh.aspx (accessed 3 October 2016).

This website has a variety of information and resources about the relationship between physical and mental health in both children and adults.

South London and Maudsley NHS (SLaM) (2015) *Physical Health and Wellbeing Handbook for Service Users and Carers*. Available at: www.slam.nhs.uk/media/253787/physical_health_and_wellbeing.pdf (accessed 3 October 2016).

This excellent booklet, written for service users and carers, describes the physical health checks that should be completed on admission to hospital for mental health care and in the year following discharge. Advice is also provided about lifestyle factors that are important in maintaining good physical health when living back in the community.

## ANSWERS TO MULTIPLE CHOICE QUESTIONS

1(d), 2(b), 3(c), 4(d), 5(d), 6(d), 7(d), 8(b), 9(b), 10(d)

# THREE

## SIGNS AND SYMPTOMS OF COMMON PHYSICAL HEALTH PROBLEMS

### PAT CONAGHAN

## CHAPTER LEARNING OUTCOMES

After reading this chapter, you will be able to:

- Identify the three most common physical health problems experienced by people with mental health problems.
- List the risk factors, presenting signs and symptoms of these conditions, as well as the impact of these conditions on a service user's physical health.
- Outline the immediate, short-term and long-term management of these conditions.

## MULTIPLE CHOICE QUESTIONS

We have included 10 multiple choice questions at the beginning of this chapter for readers wishing to test their knowledge of its contents. We have included the answers at the end of the chapter, but advise you not to check these until you have answered them before and after reading the chapter so that you can determine how much your knowledge has increased.

1. Which of the following is a non-modifiable risk factor for cardiovascular disease:

   a) Smoking.
   b) Ethnic background.
   c) Obesity.
   d) High cholesterol.

2. The commonest physical conditions experienced by people with mental health problems are:

   a) Cardiac conditions.
   b) Respiratory conditions.

*(Continued)*

*(Continued)*

    c)  Metabolic conditions.
    d)  All of the above.

3. Cardiovascular disease is the term for a number of conditions, including:

    a)  Coronary heart disease, peripheral arterial disease and cerebrovascular disease.
    b)  Coronary heart disease, cerebrovascular disease and diabetes.
    c)  Peripheral arterial disease, cerebrovascular disease and diabetes.
    d)  None of the above.

4. Common symptoms of a myocardial infarction include:

    a)  Chest pain.
    b)  Breathlessness.
    c)  Nausea.
    d)  All of the above.

5. Which one of the factors below is no longer recommended to prevent a heart attack:

    a)  Lifestyle changes, including exercise for 20–30 minutes daily.
    b)  Participating in a cardiac rehabilitation programme.
    c)  Taking omega-3 supplements.
    d)  Eating a Mediterranean-style diet.

6. Which of the following foods is *not* recommended as part of the Mediterranean diet:

    a)  Pasta.
    b)  Fish.
    c)  Fresh fruit and vegetables.
    d)  Red meat.

7. Common complications of diabetes include:

    a)  Blurred vision, pins and needles in the extremities, frequent urination.
    b)  Poor wound healing.
    c)  Difficulty breathing.
    d)  Both a and b above.

8. Which of the following are *not* part of the management of diabetes:

    a)  Lifestyle interventions, e.g. healthy diet, exercise, avoidance of alcohol and stopping smoking.
    b)  Appropriate medication, including insulin or hypoglycaemic agents intended to control blood glucose levels.
    c)  A carbohydrate free diet.
    d)  Regular assessment to prevent the development of complications, e.g. regular specialist eye checks in the form of retinopathy screening, regular foot checks.

9. Chronic obstructive pulmonary disease (COPD) is a condition that includes:

    a)  Asthma and pneumonia.
    b)  Bronchitis and asthma.
    c)  Chronic bronchitis and emphysema.
    d)  Emphysema and asthma.

10. Which of the following are recommended treatments for COPD:

    a) Eating a healthy diet.
    b) Taking regular exercise.
    c) Pulmonary rehabilitation.
    d) All of the above.

# INTRODUCTION

In this chapter, we provide an overview of the physical health problems most commonly experienced by people with mental health problems:

1. Cardiovascular disease.
2. Respiratory diseases such as COPD.
3. Metabolic disorders such as diabetes.

We outline the risk factors for these health problems and the signs and symptoms to enable early diagnosis and intervention. We will look at the impact of these conditions on the physical health and wellbeing of service users and gain an understanding of their immediate, short-term and long-term management. Please note that the advice regarding optimal management was correct at the time of writing this book, but readers should ensure that they access the most up-to-date guidance because this may change over time.

## ⚙ REFLECTION POINT 3.1

Think about service users whom you have come in contact with:

- Did you recognise that they had a physical health problem as well as a mental health problem, if so what condition did they have?
- Did you feel that you had sufficient knowledge of their condition to be able to support them?

# CARDIOVASCULAR DISEASE

'Cardiovascular disease' is the collective term for a range of conditions that affect the heart and the circulation system. Other terms you may encounter about diseases that affect the heart include 'coronary heart disease (CHD)' or 'ischaemic heart disease'; those affecting the brain are sometimes referred to as 'cerebrovascular disease'; while those affecting the rest of the body include 'peripheral vascular disease' or 'peripheral arterial disease'. Cardiovascular diseases are the biggest single cause of death in the UK, accounting for 25% of premature deaths in men and 17% in women in 2014 (Townsend et al., 2015).

## RISK FACTORS FOR CARDIOVASCULAR DISEASE

The risk factors for all forms of cardiovascular disease are listed in Table 3.1 and include both modifiable and unmodifiable elements.

Table 3.1   Risk factors for cardiovascular disease

| Modifiable | Unmodifiable |
| --- | --- |
| Smoking | Age |
| Diabetes | Ethnic background |
| High cholesterol | Family history of heart disease |
| Hypertension (high blood pressure) | |
| Obesity | |
| Physical inactivity | |

Modifiable factors are those risks that can be altered by changes in lifestyle such as quitting smoking, or by taking medications, for example statins for high choles-terol. However, some risk factors such as ethnicity, gender and age cannot be changed (see Chapter 1 for more discussion about modifiable and unmodifiable risk factors).

## SIGNS AND SYMPTOMS OF CARDIOVASCULAR DISEASE

The signs and symptoms of cardiovascular disease are listed in Table 3.2 and vary according to the area of the body affected. We begin by exploring the signs and symptoms associated with coronary heart disease.

Table 3.2   Signs and symptoms of cardiovascular disease

| Coronary heart disease | Cerebrovascular disease | Peripheral vascular disease |
| --- | --- | --- |
| Chest pain (often called angina)<br><br>Breathlessness<br><br>Pain (in the jaw, arms, upper abdomen or back)<br><br>Sweating (feeling cold and clammy) | Facial changes, including one side of the face drooping, the inability to smile, the eye appearing to droop or eyelids not open<br><br>Weakness in one side of the body in the arms or legs, with an inability to lift the limb or feelings of numbness and tingling | Painful cramping in legs or feet, often worse at night or on walking a short distance<br><br>Coldness, tingling or numbness in extremities<br><br>Discolouration of the skin or presence of slow-healing sores on the legs |

| Coronary heart disease | Cerebrovascular disease | Peripheral vascular disease |
|---|---|---|
| Seizures (may occur if the person's heart rhythm is affected) | Speech may be slurred or incomprehensible or completely absent | Men may experience erectile dysfunction |
| *Caution*: People with diabetes do not always present with severe chest pain | These symptoms may be temporary or longer lasting<br><br>(Cerebrovascular disease is discussed in more detail later) | |

## CORONARY HEART DISEASE (CHD)

Coronary heart disease (CHD) occurs as a result of the formation of atherosclerotic 'plaques' within the blood vessels supplying the myocardium (muscle of the heart). These plaques (fatty substances) reduce the space in the centre of the artery, resulting in a reduced blood flow to the heart muscle (National Heart, Lung and Blood Institute, 2016), a condition referred to as 'stable angina'. If the plaque ruptures and a blood clot forms, completely blocking the artery, the individual develops 'acute coronary syndrome', which may lead to a myocardial infarction (heart attack), cardiac arrest (heart stopping suddenly) and death.

The signs and symptoms of coronary heart disease can be mistaken for other conditions, such as panic disorder, anxiety and depression (Carleton et al., 2014). Chest pain can also be a symptom of other physical conditions, such as gastro-oesophageal reflux, costochondritis (inflammation of the cartilage in the rib cage), increased muscular tension or referred pain from the thoracic spine. It is extremely difficult to differentiate the cause of chest pain on history alone; however, the questions taken from Bass and Mayou (2002), listed in Table 3.3, can help practitioners differentiate cardiac chest pain from non-cardiac chest pain. If in any doubt of the

**Table 3.3   Questions to assess the nature of chest pain**

Questions to differentiate people with non-cardiac chest pain from those with CHD

| Question | Response | |
|---|---|---|
| | Typical | Atypical |
| If you go up a hill (or other stressor) on 10 separate occasions, on how many do you get the pain? | 10/10 | <10/10 |
| Of 10 pains in a row, how many occur at rest? | <2/10 | ≥2/10 |
| How many minutes does the pain usually last? | <5 | ≥5 |

When answers to all three questions are 'atypical', the chance of coronary disease is only 2% in people aged <55 years and 12% in those aged ≥55

If in any doubt of the diagnosis, any symptom of chest pain should be treated seriously as the consequences can be fatal

*Source*: Bass and Mayou (2002), reproduced with kind permission of BMJ Publishing Group Ltd

diagnosis, any symptom of chest pain should be treated seriously and help sought immediately as the consequences can be fatal.

---

### KEY MESSAGE 3.1

Symptoms of coronary heart disease can be confused with other conditions:

- If in doubt, seek medical help urgently.

---

## DIAGNOSIS AND MANAGEMENT OF CORONARY HEART DISEASE

The main conditions resulting from coronary heart disease are stable angina, acute coronary syndrome and heart failure. We will discuss the diagnosis and management of each of these conditions in turn.

### STABLE ANGINA

Stable angina is characterised by chest pain, precipitated by a stressor (for example, physical exercise, exposure to cold or emotional stressors) and relieved by rest or medication. The medication usually prescribed for people with stable angina is glycerol trinitrate (GTN). Stable angina is the result of the heart being unable to provide sufficient blood flow to meet the demands being placed on it because the arteries are filled with plaques (fatty substances), which limit the flow of blood to the heart.

Stable angina can usually be diagnosed by physical examination but additional diagnostic tests include non-invasive imaging such as stress echocardiography and Magnetic Resonance Imaging (MRI) as well as invasive tests such as coronary angiography.

Short-acting nitrate drugs, such as GTN, are used to prevent and treat angina episodes. People with angina will frequently take GTN prior to any event that they think may constitute a stressor. They can repeat the dose after 5 minutes but if no relief is obtained within 5 minutes of the second dose, they should call the emergency ambulance service immediately. Headaches and dizzy spells are common side effects of these drugs.

### ACUTE CORONARY SYNDROME

The term 'acute coronary syndrome' describes a number of conditions following a sudden reduction in the blood flow to the heart (Overbaugh, 2009). As described above, acute coronary syndrome occurs when the blood flow through the artery is completely blocked following the rupture of a plaque and the development of a blood clot. This may result in unstable angina, which is not resolved by rest or medication or a myocardial infarction (heart attack).

## MYOCARDIAL INFARCTION

A myocardial infarction results from the occlusion of a coronary artery that supplies the heart muscle (myocardium) with blood (Thygesen et al., 2007). Myocardial infarctions are usually graded as ST segment elevation myocardial infarction (STEMI) or Non-ST Segment Elevation myocardial infarction (NonSTEMI), depending on the degree of damage to the heart following the blockage. The ST segment is part of the normal heart rhythm, the interval between ventricular depolarisation (the electrical activity generated as the heart beats) and repolarisation (the heart preparing to beat again). The ST segment elevation myocardial infarction (STEMI) is indicative of greater damage to the heart muscle and is often life-threatening (Steg et al., 2012). A Non-ST Segment Elevation myocardial infarction (NonSTEMI), whilst still serious, usually results in less damage to the heart muscle. Both conditions require urgent action to restore the blood supply to the myocardium as over 50% of the heart muscle can be irreversibly damaged in the first hour and 75% within three hours after a myocardial infarction (Howard et al., 2015).

It is important to note that people with diabetes (discussed later in this chapter) may experience the signs and symptoms detailed above in a mild form. It is therefore essential that more in-depth testing is carried out to confirm whether they have had a myocardial infarction. At the time of writing this book, recommendations advise that a 12-lead electrocardiogram (ECG) is performed immediately. ST Segment Elevations may not be present in the early stages of a myocardial infarction, so ECGs should be repeated until a diagnosis is made. At the same time, a blood test for Troponin I or T should be taken and repeated within 10–12 hours. A rise in Troponin levels (proteins released into the blood stream when the myocardium is damaged which are used as biomarkers) indicates that a myocardial infarction has occurred.

Immediate treatment usually consists of a combination of drug therapy and removal of the clot through percutaneous coronary intervention (NICE 2013a). The aim of both treatments is to re-establish blood flow to the heart muscle.

Aspirin is one of the most important drugs in treating a myocardial infarction. Given as a single dose of 300 mg (standard tablet), it reduces the stickiness of platelets so that the blood clot cannot continue to grow. If aspirin is given before the person is sent to hospital, the hospital must be informed. Diamorphine or morphine is given as an intravenous injection to reduce stress and pain and the negative effect that these can have on the heart. One of the main side effects of opiates is nausea, therefore it is good practice to give an antiemetic such as metoclopramide at the same time. Antiplatelet drugs may also be given according to local protocols.

Oxygen should only be administered where there is evidence of hypoxia (low blood oxygen levels), pulmonary oedema (fluid on the lungs, usually seen as a pink froth in the mouth), or continuing myocardial ischaemia. Too much oxygen can be detrimental and should be avoided, especially in people with pre-existing respiratory diseases such as COPD.

Percutaneous coronary intervention is the mainstay of treatment and should take place within 90 minutes of diagnosis. This involves the introduction of a catheter into the artery and the opening of the blockage either through the use of a balloon or a stent, which will be left in place permanently. This procedure reopens the artery and restores the blood supply to the heart muscle. In order to ensure that the blood vessel does not clot a second time, people are given medication: a glycoprotein IIb/IIIa inhibitor (for example, eptifibatide) and low molecular weight heparin (for example, enoxaparin). Individuals who are not eligible for reperfusion treatments (such as a percutaneous coronary intervention) due to contraindications should be treated with low molecular weight heparin.

## LONGER-TERM MANAGEMENT OF CARDIOVASCULAR DISEASE

Individuals with any of the cardiovascular diseases should receive ongoing treatment and be encouraged to make changes to any aspects of their lifestyle that are potentially harmful.

Ongoing medication will usually consist of aspirin (75 mg). Service users should be advised not to use aspirin as a pain medicine when on low dose aspirin as the higher dose will diminish the cardio protective effect of the drug. Hypertension should be treated, usually with Acetylcholinesterase inhibitors, and all service users should be given a statin (a drug to reduce blood cholesterol levels).

The most important change in lifestyle that a person can make is to quit smoking (see Chapter 8 for advice about smoking cessation). Other changes recommended include the adoption of a healthy diet and a regular exercise regime (see Chapters 7 and 9). It is no longer advised that people take omega-3 supplements as there is little evidence of their efficacy, instead they should be advised to have two portions of fish per week. Attendance at a cardiac rehabilitation scheme (Dunlay et al., 2014) can assist people post-myocardial infarction to modify their lifestyles in line with these recommendations.

### KEY MESSAGE 3.2

Key factors for reducing risk of recurrent cardiac events include:

- Stressing the importance of lifestyle changes, including encouraging exercise for 20–30 minutes daily.
- Participating in a cardiac rehabilitation programme.

- Giving people who have had an acute myocardial infarction the right medications.
- Recommending a Mediterranean-style diet that is rich in starchy foods such as pasta, with plenty of fresh fruit and vegetables, but is low in red meat (NHS Choices, 2016b).

---

### ♟ CASE STUDY 3.1

Idrick was 52 years of age and had been diagnosed with bipolar disorder at the age of 25. He has been a heavy smoker since the age of 14. He is being treated with lithium carbonate 400 mg daily to stabilise his mood.

What potential risk factors for coronary heart disease might Idrick have?

---

# DIABETES

Diabetes is a condition in which the body's normal mechanisms for managing glucose (sugar) are damaged (Diabetes UK, 2016). Glucose is the main source of energy derived from the food we eat and is used by the cells of the body as fuel. The hormone insulin acts as a key, unlocking cells and allowing glucose to pass into them from the blood stream. When there is not enough insulin or the insulin is not functioning (that is, cannot open the door to the cells), glucose is prevented from entering the cells and remains in the blood stream. Too much glucose in the blood results in diabetes. There are three types of diabetes: type 1, type 2 and gestational diabetes.

## TYPE 1 DIABETES

Type 1 diabetes usually occurs in childhood as a result of genetics or exposure to a virus or chemicals. In type 1 diabetes, the insulin producing cells in the pancreas have been destroyed and the body cannot produce insulin. Consequently, insulin must be given as a medication via injection to make up for this.

## TYPE 2 DIABETES

Type 2 diabetes usually occurs in adulthood but can occur in children. In type 2 diabetes, the cells still produce insulin but the levels are too low or it does not work properly. Type 2 diabetes is linked to obesity (see Chapter 9), social deprivation and lack of exercise (Lindström et al., 2013).

## GESTATIONAL DIABETES

Gestational diabetes, as the name suggests, occurs during pregnancy and results from a combination of increased demands on the body and the impact of hormones produced by the placenta that increase insulin resistance. Consequently, the woman cannot produce sufficient insulin to overcome both the resistance and manage the additional demands. This leads to a build-up of glucose in the blood. Women are particularly at risk of developing gestational diabetes if they are overweight, (BMI >30), have previously delivered a large baby (4.5 kg or more), have suffered from gestational diabetes in previous pregnancies or have siblings with diabetes (Black et al., 2013). Some individuals are at higher risk due to their ethnic origin, especially those from Chinese, African-Caribbean, South Asian or Middle Eastern backgrounds (Bowers et al., 2013).

There are a number of adverse outcomes associated with gestational diabetes both for the mother and the baby. These include for the mother: the need for caesarean delivery, larger babies potentially causing more pain during birth and preeclampsia. For the baby: clinical neonatal hypoglycaemia (low blood sugar), premature delivery, shoulder dystocia or birth injury, with babies often requiring neonatal intensive care. There is also an increased risk of maternal and neonatal mortality in women with diabetes. Whilst most women find that the diabetes disappears after birth, they remain at risk of gestational diabetes in the future and a few may go on to develop type 2 diabetes. Therefore, women who suffer gestational diabetes should be carefully monitored prior to and throughout their pregnancy, in case they require ongoing care.

## SIGNS AND SYMPTOMS OF DIABETES

The main symptoms of diabetes are listed below. They are the same for all types of diabetes resulting from increased glucose in the blood:

- Urinating frequently, especially at night.
- Thirst, constant need to drink.
- Lethargy and generally feeling tired all the time.
- Weight loss not associated with dieting.
- Itching and thrush in the genital region.
- Slow-healing cuts and or wounds.
- Blurred vision.

The long-term complication of uncontrolled high blood sugar is damage to the blood vessels, consequently any area highly dependent on blood flow, especially small blood vessels, can become damaged such as the eyes, kidneys, nerves and body extremities.

## ACTIVITY 3.1    CALCULATING
## THE RISK OF DIABETES

Diabetes UK provide an excellent online resource for you to check the risk of people developing diabetes. Enter the following Diabetes UK URL into your browser and check your own risk score: https://riskscore.diabetes.org.uk/start?_ga=1.57347690.1951764267.1470138823

A diagnosis of diabetes is usually made following a physical examination and blood glucose measurements (WHO, 2016a). Blood tests include:

- A fasting blood glucose taken after a person has fasted for 8 hours.
- A glucose tolerance test, taken 2 hours after a person has been given oral glucose.
- Glycated haemoglobin (HbA1c), a test of the average blood glucose concentration over the past few weeks.

In people with diabetes, measuring HbA1c is also useful in establishing how well they are managing the condition. Diabetes is a complex disorder and there are many complications associated with it. It is important to note that type 2 diabetes may not have any direct symptoms and it may be a complication of diabetes discussed in further detail below that leads a person to seek help in the first instance.

## COMPLICATIONS OF DIABETES: HYPOGLYCAEMIA AND HYPERGLYCAEMIA

There are a number of complications that can result from diabetes. Hypoglycaemia (often referred to as a 'hypo') occurs when the level of blood sugar becomes too low to support the normal functioning of the body. The brain, in particular, is very dependent on a continuous supply of glucose and any drop in the glucose level will lead to neurological symptoms. These can come on quickly and include neurogenic (arising from the autonomic nervous system) and neuroglycopenic (resulting from glucose deprivation in the brain) symptoms. Neurogenic symptoms include shakiness, anxiety, nervousness, palpitations, sweating, dry mouth, pallor and pupil dilation. Neuroglycopenic symptoms include abnormal thinking, mood changes, confusion, aphasia, poor coordination, paresthesias, headaches, stupor and, eventually (if left untreated), seizures, coma and even death (Briscoe and Davis, 2006).

People with diabetes and their families are often aware of their own symptoms, particularly the neuroglycopenic symptoms, and can identify when a 'hypo' is occurring. Many people with diabetes carry a source of glucose with them to take in the event of a 'hypo'.

Current advice to treat a hypo in a conscious person is to give them a small glass of a sugary (non-diet) drink, some sugary sweets or glucose gel/tablets. Chocolate or snacks high in fat should not be given as the fat slows down the absorption of glucose, thus delaying recovery. Untreated hypoglycaemia can result in a loss of consciousness, therefore fast action is necessary to support the person's recovery. Oral fluids and foods should not be given to an unconscious person. Instead, they should be placed in the recovery position and the emergency services called.

Hyperglycaemia is a result of high blood sugar and may occur as a result of forgotten medication or uncontrolled diet and/or the consumption of large amounts of carbohydrate. The symptoms mirror those observed in diabetes: excessive thirst, lethargy, passing more urine than normal and headaches. Treatment includes drinking plenty of fluids and increasing insulin if required. Frequent occurrences of hyperglycaemia should be discussed with a person's treatment team because changes in their medication regime may be required.

Two emergency conditions resulting from hyperglycaemia are:

1. Hyperosmolar hyperglycaemic state: A serious condition that occurs if people become dehydrated as a result of illness or of not taking their medication. The blood sugar becomes excessively high over a period of days or weeks, which can lead to confusion, disorientation and loss of consciousness.
2. Diabetic ketoacidosis is a medical emergency. It is more common in type 1 diabetes but people with type 2 diabetes taking insulin can also develop diabetic ketoacidosis. Early symptoms of diabetic ketoacidosis include: thirst, frequent urination, feeling sick, tiredness and abdominal cramps. If left untreated, the symptoms escalate to include: confusion, drowsiness, rapid breathing, rapid heart rate, a smell of acetone (or sweet smell) on the breath. Urgent medical attention is required to return blood sugars to normal levels and prevent the development of acute kidney failure, cerebral oedema and acute respiratory distress syndrome.

## LONG-TERM COMPLICATIONS OF DIABETES

Retinopathy is damage to the blood vessels supplying the retina in the eye that can lead to partial or complete loss of vision. Regular eye screening is essential for people with diabetes to detect any early changes and prevent blindness. Other complications include:

• Neuropathy damage to the nerves which results in altered sensations such as tingling or numbness.
• Reduced sensitivity to pain or presence of burning/shooting pain, especially at night.

- Reduced sensitivity to temperature, so people may not be aware of hot surfaces and are at risk of burns and scalds.

As a result of these changes, individuals may not be aware of damage to their body, particularly the feet and a condition known as 'diabetic foot syndrome' can develop and professional foot care should be provided. Kidney disease can occur due to damage to the capillaries supplying blood to the kidneys, resulting in them becoming less efficient and ultimately leading to renal failure.

---

**👤👤👤 CASE STUDY 3.2**

Stephen is an 18-year-old student, previously under the care of the Child and Adolescent Mental Health Services (CAMHS) team and is transitioning to adult mental health services. Stephen is prescribed 300 mg of clozapine daily to treat his psychosis. As his care coordinator, you receive a call from his mother, who is concerned about changes in his behaviour. When you call round to see him, you note that he is drowsy and his breath smells sweet. On speaking with his mother, she tells you that he has been going to the toilet frequently and drinking copious amounts of water; she also tells you that he has been vomiting, has had abdominal pain and is becoming confused.

What do you think is wrong with Stephen? What action should you take?

---

## EFFECTIVE MANAGEMENT OF DIABETES

The five basic principles of diabetes management (WHO, 2016a) include:

1. Lifestyle interventions, for example healthy diet, regular exercise, avoidance of alcohol and quitting smoking.
2. Appropriate medication, including insulin or hypoglycaemic agents intended to control blood glucose levels.
3. Medication to reduce the associated risk of cardiovascular disease.
4. Regular assessment to prevent the development of complications, for example regular specialist eye checks in the form of retinopathy screening, regular foot checks.
5. Clear criteria for referral of service users from primary care to secondary care.

Immediate management of diabetes is focused on blood glucose control and the prevention of life-threatening consequences. Longer-term management is focused on maintaining blood glucose control and the prevention of complications of the condition.

# RESPIRATORY DISORDERS

## SIGNS AND SYMPTOMS OF CHRONIC OBSTRUCTIVE PULMONARY DISEASE (COPD)

Chronic obstructive pulmonary disease (COPD) is an overarching term used to describe a number of lung conditions, including chronic bronchitis and emphysema. Chronic bronchitis results from an inflammation of the air passages (bronchioles) in the lungs that causes the production of excess mucus, leading to a cough and the expectoration of a thick discoloured mucous. Emphysema occurs when the air sacs (alveoli) in the lungs become damaged; the inner walls rupture causing enlargement of the air sacs which then reduces the amount of oxygen that can cross through the lungs into the bloodstream, resulting in breathlessness.

## SYMPTOMS OF COPD

Common symptoms of COPD include:

- Shortness of breath.
- Chronic cough.
- Sputum production that can be white, yellow, green or clear.
- Blue-tinged lips or fingernails.
- Wheezing.
- Chest tightness.
- Frequent chest infections.
- Unintended weight loss.

## DIAGNOSIS AND MANAGEMENT OF COPD

The main cause of COPD is smoking. A diagnosis should be considered in people over 35 years of age who have a history of smoking and present with a chronic cough, breathlessness, regular production of sputum and a wheeze (NICE, 2008: public health guidelines (PH)15).

Diagnostic tests include spirometry, which is a common lung function test that assesses how well a person can breathe in and out. It is often used to aid diagnosis and assess the effect of treatment. Post-bronchodilator spirometry is used to confirm the diagnosis of COPD. Other diagnostic tests include chest X-rays, sputum-testing and pulse oximetry, which is a non-invasive procedure to measure oxygen levels in the blood. A full blood count helps rule out anaemia as a source of breathlessness and a computerised axial tomography (CT) scan may be carried out if other lung diseases are suspected.

The symptoms of COPD can be mistaken for asthma. Table 3.4 identifies the features from the history and examination of a person which differentiate these two conditions.

**Table 3.4 Clinical features differentiating chronic obstructive pulmonary disease (COPD) and asthma**

|  | Chronic obstructive pulmonary disease (COPD) | Asthma |
| --- | --- | --- |
| Smoker or ex-smoker | Nearly all | Possibly |
| Symptoms under age 35 | Rare | Often |
| Chronic productive cough | Common | Uncommon |
| Breathlessness | Persistent and progressive | Variable |
| Night-time waking with breathlessness and/or wheeze | Uncommon | Common |
| Significant diurnal or day-to-day variability of symptoms | Uncommon | Common |

# MANAGEMENT OF COPD

As the damage in the lungs is irreversible, treatment of COPD is aimed at managing the symptoms and slowing down the progression of the disease.

## SMOKING CESSATION

The main cause of COPD in developed countries is smoking. Anyone who develops the condition should be encouraged to stop smoking. Evidence-based approaches to support smoking cessation are discussed in detail in Chapter 8.

## LIFESTYLE CHANGES AND PULMONARY REHABILITATION

As with other conditions, lifestyle changes can improve the symptoms of COPD. Eating a healthy diet and exercise are beneficial. In some instances, service users can attend pulmonary rehabilitation, a series of exercise classes aimed at improving the strength and fitness of the lungs, providing education to support self-management of the condition and supporting them emotionally.

## INHALER THERAPY

In the first instance, short-acting inhalers are used to manage breathlessness and improve exercise tolerance. They work by dilating the bronchioles to allow more air to flow through. Longer-acting bronchodilators are available that can last up to 12 hours.

Inhaled corticosteroids are usually prescribed when the service user has repeated flare-ups of the condition. They work by reducing the inflammation in the airways. Often the two drugs are given in combination. In an acute exacerbation of COPD, inhaled bronchodilators and steroids are given via a nebuliser, which aids dispersion of the drug within the lungs.

### OXYGEN THERAPY

In some instances, the levels of oxygen in the blood remain too low, even when medication is prescribed. In these instances, service users may require supplemental oxygen. Oxygen therapy will only be prescribed once specialist assessment has been carried out. There are a number of different regimes that are tailored to the individual's needs, aimed at improving oxygen levels at different times of the day or during activity.

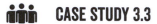 **CASE STUDY 3.3**

Edna is 62. She was diagnosed with schizophrenia in her early twenties. A lifelong smoker, she currently smokes 30 cigarettes a day. Over the past few years, she has become increasingly breathless, and has suffered what she refers to as 'winter bronchitis'. You are completing a physical health assessment of Edna: which diagnosis might you consider and what advice would you give Edna?

## CONCLUSION

Coronary heart disease, diabetes and chronic obstructive pulmonary disease are common physical health concerns for people with mental health problems. Lifestyle changes make a significant contribution to reducing the risk of developing these diseases and in managing them if they occur. Annual physical health checks should be routine for all people with mental health problems (see Chapter 10) and should include assessments for the above conditions. All people with mental health problems with risk factors for the above conditions should receive prompt treatment and support.

## USEFUL RESOURCES

British Heart Foundation website. Available at: www.bhf.org.uk.

Useful source of information and advice to professionals and patients on cardio vascular diseases.

British Lung Foundation website. Available at: www.blf.org.uk/.

Useful source of information and advice to professionals and patients on respiratory diseases.

Diabetes UK website. Available at: www.diabetes.org.uk/.

Useful source of information and advice to professionals and patients on diabetes.

NICE Pathways website. Available at: http://pathways.nice.org.uk/.

Comprehensive and easy-to-use access to all NICE guidance arranged by subject.

# ANSWERS TO MULTIPLE CHOICE QUESTIONS

1(b), 2(d), 3(a), 4(d), 5(c), 6(d), 7(d), 8(c), 9(c), 10(d)

# PRIMARY, SECONDARY AND TERTIARY PREVENTION

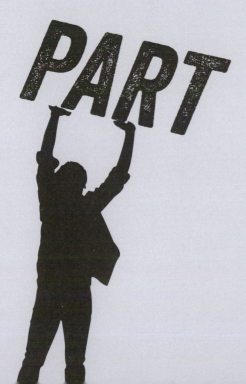 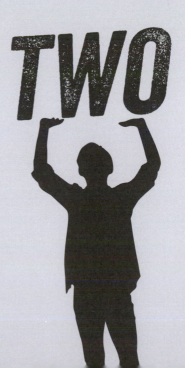

# FOUR

## ASSESSING AND MONITORING PHYSICAL HEALTH

### PAT CONAGHAN AND NIGEL HENDERSON

### CHAPTER LEARNING OUTCOMES

After reading this chapter, you will be able to:

- Understand how to conduct assessments of physiological and neurological observations.
- Understand the relevant anatomy and physiology and the concept of homeostasis.
- Be able to identify the deteriorating service user and take appropriate action.
- Be able to assess a person in a medical emergency and take appropriate action.

### MULTIPLE CHOICE QUESTIONS

We have included 10 multiple choice questions at the beginning of this chapter for readers wishing to test their knowledge of its contents. We have included the answers at the end of the chapter, but advise you not to check these until you have answered them before and after reading the chapter so that you can determine how much your knowledge has increased.

1. Homeostasis is the body's way of:

    a) Repairing damage.
    b) Staying in balance despite internal and/or external changes.
    c) Changing how an organ works.
    d) Ensuring adequate sleep.

2. Which of these parameters make up the NEWS score:

    a) Blood pressure, temperature, respiration, blood sugar, level of consciousness.
    b) Systemic blood pressure, respiratory rate, cardiac output, pulse, oxygen saturation.

*(Continued)*

*(Continued)*

    c) Respiratory rate, oxygen saturation, temperature, systolic blood pressure, pulse rate, level of consciousness, plus supplementary oxygen.
    d) Oxygen saturation, pulse rate, respiratory rate, level of consciousness, temperature.

3. The peripheral nervous system:

    a) Contains receptors that sense changes in the external environment.
    b) Contains receptors that sense changes in the internal environment.
    c) Contains receptors that sense changes in the external and internal environment.
    d) Does not contain receptor neurons.

4. The Central Nervous System:

    a) Interprets impulses from receptors.
    b) Activates effector organs such as muscles and glands.
    c) Has two divisions: the somatic and autonomic.
    d) All of the above.

5. A temperature outside of the normal range which is above 37°C is called:

    a) Hyperthermia.
    b) Normothermia.
    c) Hypothermia.
    d) None of the above.

6. A respiratory rate of 21:

    a) Is normal and raises no concerns.
    b) Is too low and medical advice should be sought.
    c) Is too high but requires no action.
    d) Is too high and medical advice should be sought.

7. A service user has a respiratory rate of 20, oxygen saturations of ≤91, a temperature of 39°C, a BP of ≤90 and a heart rate of 130. They are receiving oxygen 2l/min via nasal specs. They are confused but respond to questions you ask. Their NEWS score is:

    a) 15
    b) 13
    c) 17
    d) 12

8. In the ABCDE approach, the letters stand for:

    a) Airway, Blood pressure, Circulation, Disability, Exposure
    b) Airway, Breathing, Circulation, Disability, Environment
    c) Airway, Breathing, Circulation, Disability, Exposure
    d) Airway, Blood glucose, Capillary refill, Disability, Environment

9. In an emergency, the best assessment to use is:

    a) ABCDE.
    b) NEWS score.
    c) General Physical Health Assessment.
    d) None of the above.

10. SBAR stands for:

   a)  Situation, Background, Action, Review
   b)  Situation, Behaviour, Action, Review
   c)  Summary, Background, Assessment, Recommendation
   d)  Situation, Background, Assessment, Recommendation

# INTRODUCTION

Homeostasis is the body's system for maintaining health through a process of sending, interpreting and acting, which breaks down when disease is present. In this chapter, we explore this concept in further detail and introduce two frameworks that support health care professionals to act as external mechanisms to restore homeostasic balance. These are: (1) the National Early Warning Sign Score (Royal College of Physicians, 2012) which enables assessment and identification of the acutely ill patient to summon appropriate assistance; and (2) the ABCDE approach (Thim et al., 2012), which supports the rapid assessment of people in a medical emergency and identifies the possible cause of this and key action to take. In conclusion, we introduce an additional framework to facilitate effective communication when physical health problems are detected, the SBAR tool (Situation, Background, Assessment and Recommendation).

# HOMEOSTASIS

Physical and mental health problems are the result of physical and chemical changes in the brain and other functions that make up the body (Clancy and McVicar, 2009). The normal functioning of these systems ensures that the internal environment within which our cells exist remains constant or balanced, in spite of influences that affect our body. This balance is given the name 'homeostasis', which means 'like (homeo) standing still (stasis)', although it is a series of very active processes that ensure our cells are provided with all the materials needed to carry out their functions. When this balance is disturbed, it impacts adversely on body systems, resulting in abnormal clinical observations relating to temperature, blood glucose levels and so on. Indeed, most disease can be regarded as a breakdown in the regulation of conditions needed to maintain a homeostatic balance (Marieb and Hoehn, 2016).

## *HOW IS HOMEOSTASIS MAINTAINED?*

Homeostasis is maintained by the interaction of the central nervous system and hormones, with the central nervous system acting as a sensor and interpreter of information and hormones and the nervous system as the active agents that the body uses to restore balance. Basically, three components are required, the first being a sensor which monitors a specific aspect within a system called a 'parameter'. This sensor communicates with a specific neurological centre in the central nervous system, which interprets the sensor's measurements. If the parameter value is outside of the normal limits, then the neurological centre acts to return the measurement to within those normal limits by initiating a suitable response.

Health professionals act very much like a homeostatic mechanism, albeit an external one, when we consider that we assess and measure our service user's parameters and 'sense' the physiological and psychological measurements, we then undertake an 'interpretation' of these and plan an 'action' to treat any abnormal findings, implementing prescribed interventions, and, finally, evaluating or 'sensing' the effects to determine whether the actions taken have returned the observation parameter to an acceptable normal level (Clancy and McVicar, 2009).

---

### ⚙ REFLECTION POINT 4.1

Think about the assessments you are familiar with that indicate a change in homeostasis, for example temperature. Write down as many as you can identify, then see which ones you have missed as you read through this chapter.

---

## BACKGROUND PHYSIOLOGY

In order to understand how the body maintains homeostasis, we need to understand some basic physiological principles. The human body controls its internal balance via the interaction between the environment sensed by the peripheral nervous system and the response coordinated by the central nervous system.

### *PERIPHERAL NERVOUS SYSTEM*

The peripheral nervous system consists of receptors and nerves made up from groups of specialised cells called 'neurons'. Receptors are specialised cells that respond to stimuli in the environment, and are normally found in the sensing organs such as the eye, ear, tongue, nose and so on. Each responds to a different type of stimulation and are grouped by the stimulus to which they respond. Once a receptor is stimulated, it transmits signals along the sensory (afferent) neurones to the central nervous system (Table 4.1).

Neurons have the ability to transmit electrochemical signals to and from the brain. There are three types of neurons: sensory (afferent), motor (efferent) and

**Table 4.1  Types of receptors**

| Name | Stimulus | Location |
| --- | --- | --- |
| Proprioceptors | Movement and space | Muscles, tendons, inner ear (labyrinth) |
| Thermoreceptors | Temperature change | Skin |
| Nociceptors | Pain | Skin |
| Chemoreceptors | Chemicals | Tongue, nose, carotid body (group of cells found where the common carotid artery divides into the internal and external carotid arteries, one on each side of the neck) |
| Photoreceptors | Light | Eyes |
| Baroreceptors | Pressure changes | Blood vessels, especially the carotid body |

relay (interneurons). Sensory neurons send signals to the brain and the spinal cord from receptors in the body. Motor neurons receive signals from the brain and spinal cord and transmit them to the muscles and glands (collectively known as 'effectors'). Relay neurons form complex networks within the central nervous system to integrate the information received from sensory neurons and to direct the function of the body through motor neurons. They may also transmit signals directly from the sensory neurones to the motor neurones, resulting in a reflex action, for example pulling your hand away from a hot plate.

Bundles of neurons group together to form nerves, and there are three main types of nerves: (1) afferent nerves transmit signals from sensory neurons to the central nervous system; (2) efferent nerves transmit signals from the central nervous system to the effectors (glands and muscles); and (3) mixed nerves, found in the spinal column, allow for the two-way transmission of information between the peripheral nervous system and the central nervous system.

## CENTRAL NERVOUS SYSTEM (CNS)

The central nervous system (CNS) is made up of the brain and the spinal cord. It makes sense of the information coming from the peripheral nervous system and responds to changes in the environment, both internal and external to the body. It does this through a process previously described as sensor/receptors which are situated around the body that send messages via the afferent neurones, the central nervous system interprets the information and sends impulses along motor neurons to the effectors, which bring about an action. A simple example of this process is when we are cold: the receptor (in this case, the skin) senses the cold and sends a message to the body's thermoregulatory centre in the central nervous system, which then interprets the message and triggers a response or action, which is for us to shiver, thus creating warmth by expending energy.

## FUNCTIONAL DIVISIONS

The nervous system also has two functional divisions: the somatic or voluntary nervous system and the autonomic or involuntary nervous system. The somatic system connects the brain with muscles and sensory receptors in the skin and consciously controls responses to stimulus, and it is often referred to as the 'rest and digest' system. The autonomic system regulates the body's functions without conscious thought, for example breathing, and it is often referred to as the 'fight or flight' system.

The autonomic system is further divided into the sympathetic and parasympathetic, which act in opposition to each other. The sympathetic system can be likened to an emergency response system: it manages the response to injury by producing more energy to allow critical parts of the body to respond, for example raising the pulse rate, and shutting down non-essential parts of the body such as reducing blood flow to the gut and peripheries. The parasympathetic system has the opposite effect: it returns the body to a resting state, reducing the heart rate, increasing the blood flow to the gut to allow for digestion and returning the flow to the peripheries.

Having a basic understanding of the nervous system is essential to understanding how the clinical assessments you make reflect what is happening in the body. There are multitudes of clinical assessments that you can complete and some are referred to elsewhere in the book (Chapters 5 and 10). For the purposes of this chapter, we will focus on those assessments that are the most indicative of deterioration in a service user's condition and the level of help that you should summon to assist in managing their care.

# NATIONAL EARLY WARNING SCORE (NEWS)

The use of early warning scoring systems to address shortfalls in the recognition of and response to service users when their physical health deteriorates is recommended in a number of UK-based reports (Smith et al., 2013c). For example, the National Patient Safety Agency (2007) estimated that 11% of all deaths reported on resulted from failures to recognise or act on deteriorations in physical health. These systems allocate points in a weighted manner when a series of predetermined vital signs deviate from a specified normal range. The total of these points is then used to indicate the severity of a service user's illness and determine optimal action, whether that is to increase observation and monitoring or commence intervention. The now widely adopted National Early Warning Score (NEWS; Smith, Prytherch et al., 2013) published by the Royal College of Physicians (2012), includes the following physiological parameters:

- Respiratory rate (breaths per minute)
- Temperature (°C)
- Oxygen saturation
- Systolic blood pressure (mmHg)

- Heart/pulse rate (beats per minute)
- Level of consciousness

We will explain and outline procedures for accurate measurement for each of these parameters in turn. All measurements should be taken while the service user is resting, rather than after a period of enhanced activity. A usual pulse rate lies between 60 and 100 when resting but increases to well over 100 after a period of exercise.

## RESPIRATORY RATE

Respiratory rate is a significant indicator of acute deterioration (Royal College of Physicians, 2012) and is the parameter most closely associated with cardiac arrest and death (Cretikos et al., 2008). An elevated respiratory rate can be a sign of pain, distress, infection, central nervous system disturbance or metabolic disturbances such as ketoacidosis (refer back to Chapter 3 for definitions of these problems). The normal rate of respiration in adults is 12–20 breaths per minute. Rates of over 20 indicate acute illness and those of over 25 indicate critical illness (ibid., 2008). A low respiratory rate can be a key indicator of problems in the central nervous system or a narcotic overdose.

### MEASURING RESPIRATORY RATE

Respiratory rate is the number of breaths taken per minute. One respiration is marked by the full rise and fall of the chest, which, for accuracy, should be counted for the duration of one minute: the pattern should be regular and the depth of the breaths consistent.

Commonly used descriptions of different types of respiratory pattern include:

- Tachypnoea: A regular respiratory rate of over 20 breaths per minute.
- Bradypnoea: A regular respiratory rate of less than 12 breaths per minute.
- Dyspnoea: Shortness of breath or difficulty in breathing, examples include the Kussmauls breathing seen in severe ketoacidosis, which is characterised by deep and rapid respirations.
- Apnoea: Absence of breathing, this can be intermittent or complete and is a serious sign.
- Cheyne Stokes: Breathing is slow, shallow and with pauses that may be quite long, this is often seen in dying people.
- Agonal: Sporadic, gasping breaths, often noisy, may sound like snoring. These can be distressing to people as it appears that the service user is fighting to breathe, however they are a reflex action of the brain stem and the service user is likely to have lost consciousness, not have a pulse and be in cardiac arrest. They should not be considered active breathing or normal breathing and should be treated with rescue breaths in the case of a cardiac arrest.

## OXYGEN SATURATION (SPO$_2$)

Although a small proportion of the oxygen we breathe is dissolved in blood plasma, the majority is chemically combined with a protein called 'haemoglobin', which is found in the red blood cells. Haemoglobin is the main means of transporting oxygen around the body and is what gives blood its distinctive red colour. The control of oxygen saturation is a relatively passive process that relies on the basic principles of physics related to gases. Whilst the central nervous system does not directly influence the uptake of oxygen by the haemoglobin molecule, it does sense changes in the pressure of oxygen in the blood and can act to increase levels of oxygen by increasing the respiratory rate.

Each haemoglobin molecule can combine with up to four oxygen molecules. The haemoglobin molecule only takes up oxygen when the concentration of oxygen in the blood is high. This high concentration leads to a high partial pressure of oxygen in the blood and increases the haemoglobins affinity for oxygen. In other words, when there is a lot of oxygen available, the haemoglobin molecule will absorb as much oxygen as it can. Conversely, as blood travels to the tissues, the pressure of oxygen in the blood is much lower and this causes the haemoglobin to release the oxygen molecules into the tissue because, at lower pressures, haemoglobin cannot maintain its affinity for oxygen.

## MEASURING OXYGEN SATURATION

At any one time, it is possible to measure the percentage of haemoglobin in arterial blood, which is saturated with oxygen, the SaO$_2$. The optimal way to do this continuously and non-invasively is via pulse oximetry (often referred to as SpO$_2$), an easy and painless measure of how effectively oxygen is being carried to parts of the body furthest from the heart. A probe (clip-like device) is placed, usually on the finger. Fingers should be clean and any nail varnish removed as this can affect the absorption of the infrared light and give false readings. Probes are available for toes and ears if it is not possible to take the measurement from a finger. Service users should be advised to remain still while the measurement is taken.

The probe uses light to measure levels of oxygen in the blood, estimating the percentage of oxygenated haemoglobin. Normal levels of SpO$_2$ lie between 95% and 100%. Whilst this measure is a good proxy for SaO$_2$, it is not entirely accurate and in service users who are critically ill, SaO$_2$ measurements, via the testing of blood samples, should be made.

## TEMPERATURE

Extremes of temperature are sensitive markers of physiological disturbance and acute illness (Royal College of Physicians, 2012). The body produces heat as a by-product of metabolism, which is the production of energy used to power the muscles and organs. In order for the human body to function normally, it must maintain a consistent internal temperature. Normal body temperature should be 37°C, (+/- 1°C). At these temperatures, the human body can function properly, however any rise or fall in temperature outside this narrow range can cause problems.

Temperature can differ between the core (central organs) and the periphery (limbs), and can vary throughout the day, being lowest in the morning and highest in the evening.

Common terms associated with body temperature are:

- Normothermia: Body temperature maintained within normal range.
- Hyperthermia (>40°C): Body temperature is elevated above the normal range.
- Pyrexia (Fever) (<38.3°C): The body's response to pyrogens (substances which cause fevers).
- Hypothermia (<35°C): Body temperature is reduced to below the normal range.

## MEASURING TEMPERATURE

Normally, it is the core body temperature that is measured, whilst peripheral temperature is usually only measured where there are concerns relating to possible loss of blood supply to a limb following an accident or surgery.

The way in which temperature is measured depends on the degree of accuracy required, access to the site for recording and the type of equipment available.

A simple and accurate means of assessing temperature is to measure it orally. This may be done with a digital thermometer with a protective sleeve, or an alcohol-filled glass thermometer (usually coloured blue). Mercury glass thermometers should no longer be used due to the toxicity of mercury. The thermometer should be placed under the person's tongue, either for three minutes if using a glass thermometer or several seconds if using a digital device. The glass thermometer should be set at a temperature below 35°C prior to insertion; this is achieved by shaking the thermometer firmly. It is important to be aware that having a hot or cold drink prior to taking the temperature can affect the reading.

Tympanic thermometers measure the temperature of the membrane in the ear. They are quick and easy to use and, if used correctly, provide accurate measures of core temperature (Jefferies et al., 2011). The ear should be clear of wax or other debris, and without sign of damage. Most come with disposable covers, which are placed over the probe. The infrared sensor should cover the tympanic membrane and the ear canal should be sealed. The sensor should never be inserted into the ear. The reading should be interpreted in line with the manufacturer's instructions.

The most accurate measurement of core temperature is to take it rectally. However, due to its invasive nature, this is rarely used in adults but it is frequently used with children. The thermometer should be cleaned with soapy water or an alcohol swab and a water-based lubricant applied to the tip. It should be gently inserted and remain in place until a reading is obtained (digital) or for three minutes (glass).

Temperature may also be recorded under a person's armpit (axillary), but this method is the least accurate and is seldom used in practice.

## BLOOD PRESSURE

This is the pressure exerted by the blood against the walls of the arteries. It is highest following contraction of the heart (systolic) and is lowest when the heart is at rest (diastolic). Both measurements are recorded when measuring blood pressure, however in the context of the acutely deteriorating service user, the systolic pressure is the more important measurement as it reflects a weakening of the heart and a reduction in its ability to pump blood out to the rest of the body.

In the presence of acute illness, the most significant aspect of systolic blood pressure measurement are low or falling readings (Royal College of Physicians, 2012). Hypotension (low blood pressure) is an indication of circulatory collapse, which can be caused by a number of conditions such as sepsis, hypovolaemia or cardiac failure. Whilst hypertension (raised blood pressure) is also an indicator of ill health in the context of severe acute illness, it is less useful in identifying deterioration.

### MEASUREMENT OF SYSTOLIC BLOOD PRESSURE

Most clinical areas use digital machines to measure blood pressure, however the steps to obtaining an accurate reading are the same for manual or automatic procedures. For the purposes of the NEWS, only systolic blood pressure is measured.

Blood pressure should be measured when the arm is level with the heart and the correct cuff size should be used. Failure to do this can result in significantly inaccurate readings. The brachial artery should be identified and palpated while the arrow of the cuff points to the location of where the pulse has been taken.

If using an automatic machine, follow the manufacturer's directions. If recording a manual blood pressure, palpate the brachial artery at the antecubital fossa (crook of the arm) and place the stethoscope over it. Slowly inflate the cuff until you can no longer hear the sound of the pulse; try to avoid over-inflating the cuff as this can be uncomfortable for the service user. Slowly deflate the cuff and note the point at which the sound of the pulse returns (known as the 'Korotkoff sound'), this is the systolic blood pressure.

## PULSE RATE

Pulse rate is an assessment of the number of times the heart beats per minute. The pulse rate is another sensitive indicator of a deteriorating service user, indicating circulatory collapse or cardiac rhythm problems. A fast heart rate can be a result of sepsis, cardiac arrhythmias or hypovolaemia. In contrast, a slow heart rate may be indicative of medication cardiac rhythm disturbances or central nervous system depression (Royal College of Physicians, 2012).

Common terms used to describe different pulse rates and rhythms are:

- Sinus rhythm: Pulse rate maintained within normal range, with a regular rhythm.
- Tachycardia (>100): Pulse rate is elevated above the normal range.
- Bradycardia (<60): Pulse rate is reduced to below the normal range.

## MEASUREMENT OF THE PULSE RATE

The pulse can be measured at any place that allows an artery to be compressed against a bone, for example at the neck (the carotid artery) or the one on the inside of the elbow (brachial artery). The choice of site is determined by ease of access and the physical state of the service user.

The most common site for recording the pulse in a healthy individual is at the radial artery in the wrist. Two fingers are placed over the artery, with sufficient pressure to feel the pulsation but not too much so that the artery is occluded. Each pulsation is counted for a full minute to ensure accuracy, the strength and rhythm of the pulse should also be noted. An irregular or weak pulse can be a sign of a cardiac rhythm problem such as atrial fibrillation, which can decrease the amount of blood circulating as it does not allow the heart to fill with blood properly.

In a person who is acutely ill, the peripheral pulses such as the radial artery (wrist) may be weak or absent as the body reduces blood flow to the extremities. It is easier to feel for the major pulses such as the femoral (located in the groin) or the carotid (located in the neck). In cases where cardiac arrest is suspected, you should always try to feel for a major pulse such as the carotid.

## LEVEL OF CONSCIOUSNESS

Reduction in the level of consciousness is one of the early signs that a service user is deteriorating. A service user may be confused or answer questions inappropriately. While this could be a mental health concern, it can also be a manifestation of deteriorating physical health; therefore, any new onset of confusion should be urgently evaluated.

The Royal College of Physicians (2012) advocate the use of a simplified neurological assessment tool, the AVPU scale, to rapidly assess level of consciousness through a straightforward assessment of four responses:

Alert – the service user is awake or opens their eyes spontaneously or in response to a question.

If a service user is alert, then the brain's sensory function is normal. However, they may be confused and any new onset or worsening of confusion should be assessed and reported.

Voice – the service user gives a minimum response to your voice, but does not open their eyes spontaneously.

This is a lower level of consciousness; reasons for this should be assessed, for example is the service user taking any narcotic medication? The response may be opening the eyes, moving a limb or making a grunting noise. They are unlikely to respond with a coherent sentence.

Pain – the service user only responds to painful stimuli by withdrawing from the pain.

This is a deeper level of unconsciousness that may be due to brain injury or drugs overdose. Remember to take care when attempting to elicit a response with painful stimulus as physical injury can result. An accepted method to obtain a response is the sternal rub, the nurse's knuckles are firmly rubbed on the middle of the sternum. Service users in this state should always be urgently reviewed.

Unresponsive – the service user does not respond to voice or pain.

This is the deepest level of unconsciousness and requires immediate attention and assessment to determine cause and immediate treatment. This may be as a result of a significant head injury, metabolic disturbances such as diabetes, or overdose of recreational and/or therapeutic drugs. It is important to ensure that the service user's airway is open and, if necessary, supported.

## CALCULATING THE NEWS SCORE AND TRIGGERING HELP

In addition to the physiological parameters, a final element is added to the overall score. The use of supplemental oxygen is usually confined to service users who are already at risk of deterioration, therefore a weighted score is added for those who are receiving oxygen therapy to reflect their higher risk.

The NEWS score reflects the degree of clinical risk that the service user has for deteriorating health. The score has two elements: the aggregate score (the sum of all the parameters and the weighted score for supplemental oxygen), and single high scores. A single high score in any of the parameters should be investigated, given the problems they can indicate.

### HOW TO CALCULATE AND INTERPRET A NEWS SCORE

Each parameter should be totalled and an additional 2 points added where the service user is receiving supplemental oxygen. Individual hospitals should determine the cut-off for each of the following:

- Whether escalation of clinical care is required and its urgency.
- The competencies of the clinical review required.
- The frequency of monitoring required.
- The most appropriate setting for ongoing clinical care. (Royal College of Physicians, 2012)

### ⚙ REFLECTION POINT 4.2

- Does your ward have a NEWS policy?
- Are you aware of the different levels of response that each score should trigger?

Table 4.2 News score chart (Royal College of Physicians, 2012)

| Physiological Parameters | 3 | 2 | 1 | 0 | 1 | 2 | 3 |
|---|---|---|---|---|---|---|---|
| Respiration Rate | ≤8 | | 9–11 | 12–20 | | 21–24 | ≥25 |
| Oxygen Saturations | ≤91 | 92–93 | 94–95 | ≤96 | | | |
| Any Supplemental Oxygen | | Yes | | No | | | |
| Temperature | ≤35.0 | | 35.1–36.0 | 36.1–38.0 | 38.1–39.0 | ≥39.1 | |
| Systolic BP | ≤90 | 91–100 | 101–110 | 11–219 | | | ≥220 |
| Heart Rate | ≤40 | | 41–50 | 51–90 | 91–110 | 111–130 | ≥131 |
| Level of Consciousness | | | | A | | | V,P or U |

### 👥 CASE STUDY 4.1

Mary is 65 years old and has a diagnosis of schizophrenia. She struggles to maintain her personal hygiene and is often unkempt. Recently, she cut her leg on an old garden rake. She has been bandaging the area herself and refuses to allow anyone to treat it. Today, you see Mary and note that she is confused. You carry out a set of observations and note that her pulse is 120 at rest, she has a temperature of 39.2°C but says she feels cold and shivery. Her respiratory rate is 22. Her blood pressure is 100/70.

- What do you think her NEWS score is if her $SpO_2$ is 93% on air?
- What level of clinical competence and seniority would you want to assess Mary?

Answers at the end of the chapter.

## ASSESSMENT IN AN EMERGENCY

Assessment in an emergency needs to be rapid and identify the most serious problems to initiate appropriate treatment. Thim et al. (2012) describe the ABCDE approach as applicable in all clinical emergencies for immediate assessment and treatment. The Resuscitation Council (UK) (2015) also advocate the use of the ABCDE approach to assess deteriorating or critically ill service users:

A – Airway

B – Breathing

C – Circulation

D – Disability

E – Exposure

The ABCDE approach should be carried out in sequence; if there is any change in one of the parameters, a reassessment should occur. Following any intervention, the service user should be reassessed to determine the impact of the treatment.

## A – AIRWAY

The airway should be assessed first as an obstruction is a life-threatening event and must be treated immediately. Obstruction in unconscious people can be caused by the muscles of the tongue relaxing, resulting in it falling back or the increased risk of vomiting. In order to determine if the tongue is the cause of the obstruction or some other foreign body, it is important to move the head in such a way that the tongue is moved away from the pharynx. This is done by a simple manoeuvre: the head tilt, chin lift. To do this, one hand is placed on the person's forehead and gentle pressure applied to move the head backward. At the same time, the other hand is used to pull their chin forward and up. This pulls the tongue from the airway and normal breath sounds should then be heard. If no normal breath sounds are heard, then the airway remains obstructed and additional urgent intervention will be required to clear it.

Once the airway has been opened, the next stage is to assess breathing.

## B – BREATHING

Breathing is assessed by looking, listening and feeling for breath close to the service user's mouth whilst watching for the rise and fall of the chest. The respiratory rate should be counted if breathing is present and any abnormal or uneven movements of the chest noted. Those with the requisite training may auscultate the chest and note any decreased or absent sounds. Finally, check the position of the trachea, which should be in the midline of the chest. A deviation may indicate a pneumothorax – this is when air has entered the space between the lung and the chest wall which may interfere with normal breathing (sometimes referred to as a 'collapsed lung').

If any problems are identified, such as inadequate rate or depth or breathing, highly abnormal breathing or absence of breathing, help should be summoned immediately and appropriate steps taken to support the service user's breathing.

## C – CIRCULATION

The rate, rhythm and strength of the major pulse such as the femoral (located in the groin) or the carotid (located in the neck) should be recorded. Where the pulse is absent, the cardiac arrest team should be called immediately and cardiac compressions started.

Quickly assess peripheral circulation using Capillary Refill Time (CRT): this is done by pressing with a finger on an exposed part of the body such as the chest or fingertip. Sufficient pressure should be applied to cause blanching of the skin and it should be held for 5 seconds. Release the pressure and immediately count the number of seconds taken for colour to return to the area. Normal CRT should be less than 2 seconds, any longer than this suggests poor peripheral circulation. However, if the temperature around the service user is low or they are elderly this could be a cause of the slow CRT.

Measure the service user's blood pressure if possible. If they have no pulse as in cardiac arrest, they will not have a blood pressure.

Where possible, attach the service user to a cardiac monitor so that the heart rhythm can be assessed directly.

## D – DISABILITY

The AVPU scale (Alert, Pain, Voice, Unresponsive) can be used to rapidly assess level of consciousness. In addition, the service user's pupil reactions should be assessed: this is done by asking them to open both eyes, you then assess the size of the pupils to see if they are abnormally dilated or constricted, and then test for their reaction to light using a pen torch shone onto the eye from one side. In a healthy individual, both eyes should react to the light at the same time. Changes of pupil reaction, shape and size are late signs of raised pressure in the skull and should be treated as a neurological emergency. However it should be noted that it is not uncommon for healthy people to have pupils of unequal size and certain medication such as opiates, fentanyl, barbiturates can cause very small pupils (1–2 mm) and the use of eye drops such as atropine can dilate pupils.

Now is a good time to check the blood glucose level as low blood glucose can cause unconsciousness.

## E – EXPOSURE

A head-to-toe examination of the service user should be completed, including whether their peripheries are warm or cold, whether there are any obvious injuries or bleeding and whether the service user has a rash.

This brief assessment can give detailed information about the service user's physical condition. Any life-threatening injuries should be treated immediately but a full assessment should be made, even when you think that you may have identified the main problem, for example cardiac arrest, as the cause of the problem may not become apparent until you have completed the full assessment or electrocution may only be obvious from history and the presence of a small burn.

# EFFECTIVE COMMUNICATION

It is critical that teams communicate effectively when working with people when their physical health is deteriorating. The Situation, Background, Assessment, Recommendation (SBAR) technique (Leonard et al., 2004) is frequently used to structure the process.

SBAR offers a straightforward way to convey information about the deteriorating person to colleagues involved in their care. Below, we have illustrated an example of the use of the SBAR technique in relation to the care of Mary, the service user described earlier in Case Study 4.1:

- Situation: Describe what is happening, e.g. Mary, who has deteriorated and has a NEWS score of 9.
- Background: What are the circumstances leading up to this situation? E.g., Mary recently developed a wound to her leg, which is now inflamed and oozing pus. Mary has not accessed any medical care for her wound.
- Assessment: What do you think the problem is? E.g., based on the observations and the wound, you think Mary may have sepsis?
- Recommendation: What should we do to correct the problem? E.g., Mary needs to be transferred to the Accident and Emergency Department immediately.

## CONCLUSION

Conducting accurate observations of vital signs, such as recordings of respiratory rate temperature, oxygen saturation, blood pressure, pulse rate and level of consciousness as outlined in the NEWS guidelines (Royal College of Physicians, 2012), is an important part of the role of all health care practitioners. As, too, is the ability to interpret the findings of these observations and to act on them appropriately, particularly in the case of service users whose health is rapidly deteriorating. In this chapter, we described the function of homeostasis, the processes by which the body maintains its normal healthy balance and functioning and we introduced two frameworks (NEWS and ABCDE) that may be used to assess (sense) whether that balance is being maintained. We have also described an approach (SBAR) for communicating information about these observations quickly and accurately (interpret and act) to colleagues in emergency situations.

## ANSWERS TO MULTIPLE CHOICE QUESTIONS

1(b), 2(c), 3(c), 4(d), 5(a), 6(d), 7(a), 8(c), 9(a), 10(d)

## ANSWERS TO CASE STUDY 4.1

- What do you think her NEWS score is if her SpO2 is 93% on air? Answer: 13.
- What level of clinical competence and seniority would you want to assess Mary? Answer: high risk.

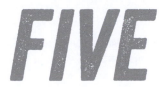

# FIVE

## PHYSICAL HEALTH OF YOUNG PEOPLE AT HIGH/ULTRA-HIGH RISK FOR PSYCHOSIS

### REBEKAH CARNEY AND JOSEPH FIRTH

## CHAPTER LEARNING OUTCOMES

After reading this chapter, you will be able to:

- Explain how we can identify young people at ultra-high risk for psychosis.
- Describe the physical health and lifestyle behaviours observed in ultra-high risk individuals.
- List the factors that affect physical health and lifestyle of ultra-high risk individuals.
- Consider the clinical implications of an unhealthy lifestyle.
- Explore options for physical health promotion for ultra-high risk individuals.

## MULTIPLE CHOICE QUESTIONS

We have included 10 multiple choice questions at the beginning of this chapter for readers wishing to test their knowledge of its contents. We have included the answers at the end of the chapter, but advise you not to check these until you have answered them before and after reading the chapter so that you can determine how much your knowledge has increased.

1.  What is the criterion for an ultra-high risk diagnosis?

    a)  Brief intermittent psychotic symptoms that spontaneously resolve.
    b)  Presence of attenuated psychotic symptoms.
    c)  Genetic risk combined with drop in functioning.
    d)  Any of the above.

*(Continued)*

*(Continued)*

2. According to a recent meta-analysis, how many times more likely were ultra-high risk individuals to smoke than their peers?

     a) 1.2
     b) 1.8
     c) 2.3
     d) 4.2

3. What did Di Forti et al. (2009) find that increased the risk of psychosis?

     a) Watching too much TV.
     b) Playing video games.
     c) Smoking high-potency cannabis.
     d) Using e-cigarettes.

4. Compared with their peers, ultra-high risk individuals are more likely to:

     a) Engage in sedentary behaviour.
     b) Be more inactive.
     c) Report more barriers to exercise.
     d) All of the above.

5. The BMI of ultra-high risk individuals compared with their peers is:

     a) No different.
     b) Lower.
     c) Slightly higher.
     d) Much higher.

6. Kumari and Postma (2005) propose that people with psychosis have higher rates of substance use because they are attempting to cope with psychological symptoms. This is:

     a) The self-medication hypothesis.
     b) The symptom-relief hypothesis.
     c) The theory of self-regulation.
     d) The theory of substance use and coping.

7. How can physical health promotion help ultra-high risk individuals?

     a) Prevent transition or worsening of mental health.
     b) Prevent future ill health.
     c) Improve overall health and wellbeing.
     d) All of the above.

8. What did Koivukangas et al. (2010) find in their longitudinal study of exercise and young people's health?

     a) Individuals who developed psychosis had lower physical activity levels during adolescence than those who did not develop psychosis.
     b) Individuals who developed psychosis had higher physical activity levels during adolescence than those who did not develop psychosis.
     c) Individuals who developed psychosis had the same physical activity levels during adolescence as those who did not develop psychosis.
     d) None of the above.

9. According to Deighton and Addington (2013), one of the barriers to taking regular exercise reported by ultra-high risk individuals was:

   a) Not having gyms in the areas where they live.
   b) Feeling tired all the time.
   c) Anxiety when exercising.
   d) Not having the appropriate clothing.

10. How can you follow the principles of 'Make Every Contact Count'?

   a) Ensure each session lasts the maximum time allowed.
   b) Use every contact as an option to discuss health promotion.
   c) Not mention health promotion unless asked by the client.
   d) Discuss as many different health issues as possible.

# INTRODUCTION

This chapter focuses on the physical health of young people at high or ultra-high risk of psychosis. We will examine evidence to suggest that young people at high/ultra-high risk of psychosis have higher rates of behavioural health risk factors for poor physical health than others their own age, even prior to the onset of psychosis. Prevention strategies that might help to promote better mental and physical health and wellbeing in this group will also be discussed.

# THE ULTRA-HIGH RISK STATE

## IDENTIFYING YOUNG PEOPLE AT ULTRA-HIGH RISK FOR PSYCHOSIS

The ultra-high risk state, also known as the 'clinical-high risk' and 'at-risk mental state' (Fusar-Poli et al., 2013), allows individuals in the prodrome for psychosis to be identified (Yung and McGorry, 1996). If you work in youth or adolescent mental health services, you may be familiar with the diagnostic tools used to establish at-risk criteria. For those less familiar, help-seeking individuals are often assessed using semi-structured interviews such as the Comprehensive Assessment of At-Risk Mental States (CAARMS; Yung et al., 2005). Measures such as the CAARMS have been shown to have excellent prognostic accuracy for detecting the ultra-high risk phase in help-seeking individuals (Fusar-Poli et al., 2015a).

In order to meet ultra-high risk criteria, an individual must have one or more of the following: presence of attenuated (subthreshold) psychotic symptoms (APS), brief limited intermittent psychotic symptoms that spontaneously resolve (BLIPS), or a genetic risk combined with a reduction in functioning (Yung et al., 2004). If left untreated, approximately 30% of individuals meeting the criteria will transition to a full-threshold psychotic disorder within three years (Nelson et al., 2013; Yung et al., 2003). In those who do not develop a psychotic disorder, many continue to experience other mental health difficulties and may be diagnosed with anxiety, mood or substance use disorders (Addington et al., 2011) and function poorly, regardless of symptoms (Cotter et al., 2014).

## EARLY DETECTION SERVICES

Young people with emerging psychological difficulties often present to mental health services with high levels of distress and poor levels of functioning. Early detection services accept young people who have had unusual experiences but do not meet the threshold for psychosis. Referrals may come from a General Practitioner (GP) or other primary care source, Child and Adolescent Mental Health Service (CAMHS), school counsellors, family members or sometimes individuals may self-refer directly to the service.

Young people should be offered support according to NICE (2014a: CG5) guidelines for the treatment of psychosis and schizophrenia in children and young people. Anyone experiencing transient or attenuated psychotic symptoms should be offered individual cognitive behavioural therapy, with or without the option of family interventions and any other treatments recommended for young people with anxiety disorders or depression. The guidelines also state that antipsychotic medication should not be offered if their symptoms do not reach the threshold for psychosis, nor should medication be offered to reduce the risk for psychosis. However, there are some cases where young people are prescribed antipsychotic medication, in low doses (McGorry et al., 2002; van der Gaag et al., 2013). Individuals who do meet criteria for a first episode of psychosis are usually referred to an early intervention for psychosis service.

---

### ⚙ REFLECTION POINT 5.1

Think about the impact of prescribing antipsychotic medication to young people. Do you agree with the NICE (2014a: CG5.8.3.2) recommendations that medication should not be offered to young people experiencing subthreshold symptoms of psychosis?

---

## EARLY IDENTIFICATION

Some people argue that identifying and labelling young people as being 'at-risk for psychosis' may be stigmatising, given that approximately 70% will not go on to experience psychosis. However, research suggests that early detection services help people cope with the self-stigma associated with experiencing mental health difficulties at an early age (Uttinger et al., 2014). Identifying people in the ultra-high risk phase is considered beneficial in a number of ways:

- Psychological therapy can minimise distress experienced during early stages of illness (Addington and Haarmans, 2006).
- Intervening during the at-risk phase can help prevent or delay the onset of psychosis, with psychological therapies such as cognitive behavioural therapy having promising results (Stafford et al., 2013; van der Gaag et al., 2013).
- Support from early detection services can have a positive impact on long-term outcome. For example, individuals with first-episode psychosis who present for treatment in early detection services often display better long-term outcome than those who do not, including fewer hospital admissions (Fusar-Poli et al., 2015b).
- Physical and psychological health of young people can be monitored prior to the onset of psychosis, providing a unique opportunity for early intervention to improve physical health.

In summary, individuals at ultra-high risk for psychosis can be identified using measures such as the CAARMS. Young people experiencing transient or attenuated psychotic symptoms should be offered cognitive behavioural therapy, with or without the option of family intervention. Antipsychotic medication is not recommended for young people in the ultra-high risk phase. Early detection and intervention is important to reduce distress, prevent or delay the onset of psychosis and improve long-term outcome.

# RISK FACTORS FOR POOR PHYSICAL HEALTH

As discussed in Chapter 3, the physical health of people with long-term mental health problems is often poor, largely because of the consequences of developing a mental health problem, the effects of medication, adverse health behaviours and the limited ability of services to respond holistically to this population. Although young people at-risk for psychosis are not usually prescribed antipsychotic medication, they do experience these other risk factors for poor physical health.

## *MONITORING OF PHYSICAL HEALTH*

Early detection services generally focus on reducing distress resulting from psychological symptoms and preventing transition to psychosis. The physical health of young people is not routinely assessed (Carney et al., 2015). There are no current guidelines to suggest that this monitoring should occur, even though we are becoming increasingly aware of the importance of monitoring physical health in service user groups, certainly in those who are at risk of co-morbid illness.

Yet, it is in these early stages that young people should be asked about their lifestyle and physical health. It is often the first time they have presented to mental health services, and represents the earliest opportunity to intervene to prevent future ill health. Nurses and other mental health professionals may be the most appropriate people to discuss physical health with young people. They are uniquely placed in the care of young people who use mental health services, with many having frequent, even daily, contact. They usually build up a relationship of trust with young people and often have a strong therapeutic alliance. In addition, nurses make up the largest component of the health care work force, resulting in an increased chance of implementation.

---

### ⚙ REFLECTION POINT 5.2

Think about young people who use mental health services:

- How might poor monitoring of lifestyle factors and physical health conditions affect their long-term health?
- Make a list of what you think should be assessed on entry to a mental health service.
- Who do you think should be responsible for collecting this information?

---

## LIFESTYLE FACTORS

There is a growing body of literature discussing the physical health and lifestyle of young people at-risk for psychosis. First, we will consider how young people with emerging psychological difficulties may be putting themselves at risk for poor physical health by engaging in unhealthy lifestyle behaviours. If you work in youth or adolescent mental health services, you may have noticed the impact that an unhealthy lifestyle can have. You may have even had discussions with young people about the effects of an unhealthy lifestyle. For those of you who may be unfamiliar with young people and adolescent mental health, some of the behaviours to consider have been illustrated in Figure 5.1.

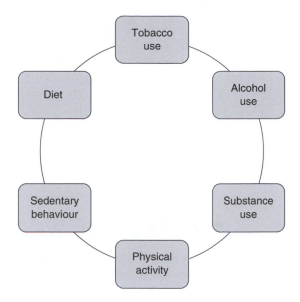

**Figure 5.1   Lifestyle factors affecting the physical health of young people**

## TOBACCO USE

A recent meta-analysis of 15 studies (Carney et al., 2016) found that approximately 33% of ultra-high risk individuals smoked, compared to only 19% of people in the general population. So, ultra-high risk individuals are 2.3 times more likely to smoke than healthy controls (see Chapter 8 for further detail regarding the prevalence of smoking). Other studies have also shown that ultra-high risk individuals smoke more heavily and consume more cigarettes per day compared with non-ultra-high risk controls (Auther et al., 2012; Huber et al., 2014).

## SUBSTANCE USE

There is a large body of evidence looking at the relationship between substance use and psychosis. Cannabis use has been shown to increase the risk of psychosis, with the greatest risk being in people using high-potency cannabis on a daily basis (Di Forti et al., 2014), or using cannabis from an early age (Dragt et al., 2012). Addington et al. (2014) found that cannabis was frequently used by ultra-high risk individuals, with rates of between 33% and 54%. The use of substances other than cannabis and alcohol is low. Yet, for many ultra-high risk individuals, substance use often progresses to a clinical problem, with many receiving co-morbid substance abuse or dependence diagnoses. It is therefore important to intervene early, perhaps by signposting to substance misuse services.

## PHYSICAL ACTIVITY AND SEDENTARY BEHAVIOURS

Ultra-high risk individuals are less likely to engage in physical activity than other young people their own age (Deighton and Addington, 2013; Hodgekins et al., 2015; Koivukangas et al., 2010; Mittal et al., 2013). They are more likely to spend their time engaging in low-intensity or sedentary activity, such as sitting at home and watching TV. Ultra-high risk individuals are therefore less likely to engage in the recommended amounts of daily exercise (see Chapter 7 for details regarding recommended amounts of daily exercise).

---

### 👥 CASE STUDY 5.1

Ryan is a 17-year-old, living at home with his parents. Ryan used to play football with his friends, however he became increasingly withdrawn and now spends a lot of time at home watching TV. Ryan reports feeling paranoid when going out, and thinks that everyone is looking at him. He also suffers from low mood and he feels like he has no energy to exercise, so he prefers to stay at home at his computer. Ryan no longer plays football with his friends because he feels like they will all watch him and will laugh at him for being unfit.

- What impact do you think Ryan's symptoms might have on his daily functioning?
- How do you think Ryan's symptoms affect his physical health?
- Can you think of any approaches that you use that might help to improve Ryan's health and wellbeing?

---

## DIET

Ultra-high risk individuals have also been shown to have poor diets, consuming significantly more calories per day than non-ultra-high risk individuals (Labad et al., 2015), suggesting that they may make poor dietary choices, although further research is needed in this area.

---

### ⚙ REFLECTION POINT 5.3

Think about any contact you may have had with young people who use mental health services. Consider their lifestyles, for example their diet, exercise levels, smoking, substance use and how healthy they are generally. Do you think that there are any differences between the health profiles of these service users and other young people you know?

## PHYSICAL HEALTH

Several markers of physical health have been discussed in previous research, and this section contains a summary of some key indicators of physical health as illustrated in Figure 5.2.

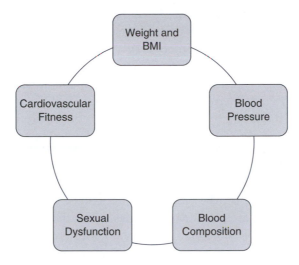

**Figure 5.2   Measures of physical health**

### WEIGHT, BODY MASS INDEX AND BLOOD PRESSURE

Anthropometric measurements, that is height, weight and blood pressure, do not seem to differ between ultra-high risk individuals and their peers (Carney et al., 2016). One reason for this may be that the majority of ultra-high risk individuals are not yet taking antipsychotic medication, and so are not exposed to the metabolic side effects which contribute to weight gain in the early stage of treatment (see Chapter 6 for more detail).

### LIPIDS AND BLOOD COMPOSITION

Identifying the blood composition of ultra-high risk individuals is important as it provides a baseline metabolic measure if they are later prescribed antipsychotic medication. The growing interest in using polyunsaturated fatty acids as an alternative treatment requires the screening of blood composition. In an ultra-high risk sample, previously increased triglyceride levels are reduced by a 12-week trial of polyunsaturated fatty acid supplements (Mossaheb et al., 2015). Therefore, we can see that there may be metabolic differences in ultra-high risk individuals, prior to being given this treatment.

## SEXUAL DYSFUNCTION

Sexual dysfunction is common in people with psychosis (de Boer et al., 2014). One explanation is that antipsychotic medication raises the levels of the hormone prolactin. However, other factors may also contribute, such as the effects of symptoms on mood, self-confidence and energy levels. Marques et al. (2012) found that sexual dysfunction occurred in 50% of ultra-high risk and 65% of first-episode psychosis, compared with 21% in healthy controls. Also, sexual dysfunction was related to symptom severity, and those who transitioned had more pronounced sexual dysfunction. One explanation could be that sexual dysfunction is driven by reduced levels of expression and activity observed in psychosis (see Chapter 11 for more information about these common problems which are often referred to as negative symptoms). Therefore, young people might benefit from discussing their sexual heath with a health professional.

## CARDIOVASCULAR FITNESS

Cardiorespiratory fitness can be assessed using a VO2 sub-max cycle-ergometer test, where people cycle at increasing intensities whilst their breathing metabolites are monitored. A large birth cohort study found no difference in cardiorespiratory fitness of adolescents when they were grouped according to levels of prodromal symptoms, or whether they developed psychosis (Koivukangas et al., 2010). However, a separate study found ultra-high risk individuals perceived themselves as having lower fitness than their peers (Deighton and Addington, 2013).

In summary, research shows that ultra-high risk individuals are more likely to engage in unhealthy behaviours such as smoking, physical inactivity and cannabis use than their peers. There is also emerging evidence regarding other physical health disparities such as sexual dysfunction, and increased triglyceride levels. However, the body mass index is often no different than their peers', suggesting that the high levels of obesity observed in people with first-episode psychosis are the result of side effects of antipsychotic medication.

## WHY DO PEOPLE AT ULTRA-HIGH RISK OF PSYCHOSIS HAVE UNHEALTHY LIFESTYLES?

As research in this area is in its infancy, we can only speculate why young people at-risk for psychosis are prone to engage in unhealthy lifestyle behaviours. However, we will briefly review three main issues that early stage research suggests may be of significance.

## PSYCHOLOGICAL FACTORS

Young people may experience more psychological barriers to engaging in healthy behaviours. For example, low mood and anxiety may deter a young person from engaging in physical activity. Ultra-high risk individuals also have reduced levels of expression and activity, often losing the ability to anticipate that they enjoy activities, which could prevent them from playing sports or exercising. Subthreshold symptoms and stigma might discourage a young person from engaging in a healthy active lifestyle. For example, they may feel more self-conscious if they exercise outdoors, or they may avoid large groups of people.

Young people at-risk for psychosis have reported significantly more barriers to exercise than controls, such as anxiety when exercising ('I do not like how my body looks') and a lack of knowledge about how to exercise (Deighton and Addington, 2013). Ultra-high risk individuals also reported fewer positive reasons to exercise, and healthy controls were more likely to agree with statements such as 'Exercise makes me healthier' and 'I will feel better about myself' than those with ultra-high risk.

## SELF-MEDICATION HYPOTHESIS

Ultra-high risk individuals may use substances to cope with psychological symptoms such as stress and anxiety. This is known as the self-medication hypothesis (Kumari and Postma, 2005). For example, ultra-high risk individuals report enhancement in mood as being the primary reason for using cannabis (Gill et al., 2013).

## SHARED RISK FACTORS

An alternative hypothesis is to consider shared risk factors for unhealthy lifestyles and psychological symptoms. For example, people who live in deprived areas are more likely to suffer poor physical and mental health (O'Donoghue et al., 2015). Unhealthy behaviours such as physical inactivity, poor diet and tobacco use are also more prevalent in young people who live in less affluent areas (Hanson and Chen, 2007). Similarly, childhood adversity contributes to the risk for psychosis, and the rates of substance use are also higher in people who have experienced adversity (Dube et al., 2003; Varese et al., 2012). Therefore, in some cases, a combination of shared risk factors may explain the high rates of unhealthy lifestyles of ultra-high risk individuals.

## ⚙ REFLECTION POINT 5.4

- Can you think of any other reasons why young people at-risk for psychosis may engage in unhealthy lifestyle behaviours?
- What barriers do ultra-high risk individuals experience and are they different from young people who do not use mental health services?

# PHYSICAL HEALTH PROMOTION FOR ULTRA-HIGH RISK INDIVIDUALS

So far in this chapter, we demonstrated that young people with emerging psychological difficulties often lead lifestyles that are less healthy than those of their peers. If ignored, this can have potential negative consequences on their physical and mental health and wellbeing, including:

- Increased risk of cardiovascular disease.
- Increased risk of ill health and co-morbid conditions.
- Negative impact on mental health and wellbeing.
- Reduced social and occupational functioning.
- Increased risk of metabolic disturbances if an individual transitions to psychosis.
- Poorer quality of life.

However, it is important to note that these behaviours are modifiable. Ultra-high risk individuals may be amenable to lifestyle interventions, such as smoking cessation programmes which may have a positive effect on both their mental and physical health (smoking cessation techniques will be described in detail in Chapter 8), and it is in this phase where mental health professionals should start to promote physical health in young people.

High rates of behavioural risk factors contribute to the risk of future ill health. Given the physical health disparities of people with serious mental illness, any pre-morbid cardiometabolic risk factors should be addressed at the earliest stage. Although not all individuals will transition to psychosis, many will continue to use mental health services. Therefore, early intervention to promote physical health in this group should be a priority.

## HOW CAN PHYSICAL HEALTH PROMOTION HELP?

Figure 5.3 illustrates some of the possible interventions that might be made to promote a healthy lifestyle and have the potential to improve physical health, mental health and wellbeing in ultra-high risk individuals.

## PREVENT TRANSITION TO PSYCHOSIS OR WORSENING OF MENTAL HEALTH

Encouraging young people who use mental health services to become more active may prevent or delay the onset of psychosis. For example, a large study found that individuals who engaged in high levels of physical activity during adolescence were less likely to have psychosis when they were assessed several years later than those

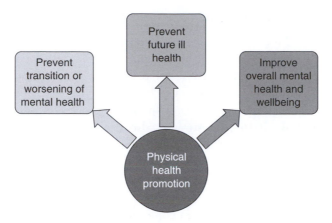

**Figure 5.3    Intervention to promote health in people at ultra-high risk of psychosis**

who were inactive (Koivukangas et al., 2010). Other research has looked at omega-3 fatty acids as a potential treatment for the UHR group, having some promising results (Amminger et al., 2015). Therefore, encouraging young people to be more active and to eat a healthy diet may exert a neuroprotective effect.

Smoking cessation and substance use interventions may also help the prognostic outcome of young people at-risk for psychosis. Both tobacco and cannabis use are thought to increase the risk of psychosis (Di Forti et al., 2014; Gurillo et al., 2015). Therefore, providing brief advice or signposting to other services may have long-term benefits.

---

### ⚙ REFLECTION POINT 5.5

Think about what might help young people to stop smoking, or dissuade them from starting smoking. How might these methods differ from those used for older adults?

---

## PREVENT FUTURE ILL HEALTH

Living an unhealthy lifestyle has a serious impact on physical health. Physical inactivity is ranked as the fourth leading cause of mortality in the general population and significantly contributes to the risk of cardiovascular disease (see Chapter 7 for more detail). Living a sedentary lifestyle also increases the risk of metabolic disease (Owen et al., 2010). Additionally, tobacco use is a major risk factor for cardiovascular disease, contributing to coronary heart disease, stroke and other major illness (WHO, 2009). We know that ultra-high risk individuals are more likely to smoke than their peers and to live a sedentary lifestyle. Therefore, encouraging people to live an active, healthy lifestyle could reduce the risk of metabolic ill health in the future.

## IMPROVE OVERALL MENTAL HEALTH AND WELLBEING

The benefits of exercise for mental health and wellbeing are well known. NICE (2010: CG1.4.2.4) recommend exercise for people with mild to moderate depression and mood disorders. Exercise has also been found to be acceptable and useful for people with first-episode psychosis, helping to reduce symptoms and improve wellbeing (Firth et al., 2016a; the study is also described in detail in Chapter 7). Alongside this, promoting a healthy diet may be beneficial. Eating a nutrient-rich diet, low in saturated fat and processed sugars, could improve overall wellbeing. In the general population, eating 5-a-day fruit and vegetables is associated with a reduction in psychological distress (Richard et al., 2015). Given the high rate of psychological distress of many young people presenting to mental health services, improvements to diet and activity could be a feasible way of promoting wellbeing.

## INTERVENTIONS TO PROMOTE PHYSICAL HEALTH AND WELLBEING

We know that interventions to improve physical health are feasible and effective in young people with psychosis (Firth et al., 2016a), and people with depression (Cooney et al., 2013). Therefore, we should be exploring how we can best work with young people to help improve their lifestyle. Some potential targets for interventions to improve physical health include:

- Smoking cessation
- Exercise promotion
- Dietary interventions to increase consumption of fruit and vegetables
- Dietary interventions to decrease fat and sugar intake
- Alcohol reduction
- Drug interventions
- Weight loss promotion
- Increased cardiovascular fitness

---

⚙️ **REFLECTION POINT 5.6**

Think about your current role:

- How can you help young people improve their physical health and live an active, healthy lifestyle?
- Make a list of the benefits that physical health promotion can have for young people at-risk for psychosis.

Happell et al. (2011) argue that more research is required in order to facilitate the integration of care for physical and mental health needs. One way of doing this is to equip mental health nurses with the necessary skills and training to conduct physical health assessments and apply interventions. Often, in your role as a mental health practitioner, it is not feasible to allocate the time and resources to developing a full-scale intervention. However, talking to people about their physical health and lifestyle can be useful. A plausible approach is training mental health practitioners to adopt the principles of 'Make every contact count' (Lawrence et al., 2016; also see Reflection Point 5.7). Here, every contact with a person is treated as a time to promote behaviour change. You could provide very brief advice to people who are struggling with their physical health or lifestyle (see Chapter 8 for more detail about very brief advice). For example, you could make young people aware of smoking cessation services in the local area. Young people may value this approach and appreciate having someone to discuss their physical health with, and whom they trust and have built up a relationship with.

---

### ⚙ REFLECTION POINT 5.7 MAKING EVERY CONTACT COUNT (MECC)

Making every contact count or MECC is recommended to encourage practitioners to help people make positive long-term changes to their lifestyle. Each contact should be seen as an opportunity to discuss lifestyle issues and explore changes that an individual wants to make. This can be stopping smoking, eating healthily, maintaining a healthy weight, reducing alcohol consumption or exercising regularly. (NHS Choices, 2016)

*Think*: Think about the conversations you have with service users. Do you make every contact count? What can you do to promote physical health in your current role?

---

## CONCLUSION

Ultra-high risk individuals display many risk factors for future ill health. The physical health and lifestyle of these young people is often poorly monitored in services and is not addressed until it becomes a clinical problem. Yet, the ultra-high risk phase represents an opportunity to promote physical health, which could also benefit mental health and overall wellbeing. Mental health practitioners are well placed to discuss behaviour change with young people. Even in those ultra-high risk individuals who do not go on to experience psychosis, lifestyle interventions can be helpful and improve other co-morbid symptoms such as depression.

## USEFUL RESOURCES

Australian Child and Young Health Network website. Available at: www.cyh.com/SubDefault.aspx?p=160.

This useful website provides a wide variety of information about health issues, lifestyle choices and relationships, and was developed specifically for young people.

NHS Choices offers a range of resources to help people move from having sedentary lifestyles to developing regular exercise patterns and losing weight:

12-week fitness plans. Available at: www.nhs.uk/Livewell/fitness/Pages/12-week-fitness-plan.aspx (accessed 3 October 2016).

Couch to 5K. Available at: www.nhs.uk/LiveWell/c25k/Pages/couch-to-5k.aspx (accessed 3 October 2016).

Healthy eating. Available at: www.nhs.uk/livewell/healthy-eating/Pages/Healthyeating.aspx (accessed 3 October 2016).

Increasing fitness. Available at: www.nhs.uk/livewell/fitness/Pages/Fitnesshome.aspx (accessed 3 October 2016).

## ANSWERS TO MULTIPLE CHOICE QUESTIONS

1(d), 2(c), 3(c), 4(d), 5(a), 6(a), 7(d), 8(a), 9(c), 10(b)

# SIX

## PROTECTING THE CARDIOVASCULAR AND METABOLIC HEALTH OF PEOPLE EXPERIENCING PSYCHOSIS FOR THE FIRST TIME

### DAVID SHIERS

## CHAPTER LEARNING OUTCOMES

After reading this chapter, you will be able to:

- Discuss why the early phase of psychosis may be a key time for preventing future life-restricting and life-shortening physical comorbidities.
- Describe how a number of potentially modifiable cardiovascular and metabolic risk factors might be targeted for intervention from the onset of psychosis and its treatment.
- Feel more confident in supporting a person experiencing psychosis for the first time in order to avoid future poor health from cardiovascular disease (CVD) and diabetes.

## MULTIPLE CHOICE QUESTIONS

We have included 10 multiple choice questions at the beginning of this chapter for readers wishing to test their knowledge of its contents. We have included the answers at the end of the chapter, but advise you not to check these until you have answered them before and after reading the chapter so that you can determine how much your knowledge has increased.

1. NICE guidelines for psychosis and schizophrenia recommend that (2014a: CG178, CG155):

*(Continued)*

*(Continued)*

a) The secondary care team should maintain responsibility for monitoring the service user's physical health and the effects of antipsychotic medication for at least the first 12 months or until the person's condition has stabilised, whichever is longer.
b) There is no specific recommendation to monitor physical health.
c) Physical health monitoring is required only for patients taking antipsychotic medication.
d) Primary care has lead responsibility for monitoring physical health from the onset of treatment.

2. Weight gain for people with their first episode of psychosis:

a) Is inevitable and best not discussed until psychotic symptoms have settled.
b) 20% gain over 7% body weight within the first 12 months of treatment.
c) Is likely to be greater for younger people taking olanzapine than other second-generation antipsychotics.
d) Less likely for those with a low BMI prior to commencing antipsychotic medication.

3. Metabolic disturbance:

a) Is evident in two-thirds of people within 8 months of starting treatment with antipsychotic medication.
b) Is invariably related to weight gain in people treated with antipsychotics.
c) Metabolic syndrome is twice as likely in people experiencing schizophrenia by age 40, compared with age-matched peers without schizophrenia.
d) With less than 7 weeks' exposure to antipsychotics, Correl et al. (2014) found rates of dyslipidemia similar to a general population averaging twenty years older.

4. According to Carney et al. (2016), compared to peers without psychiatric difficulties, people at high risk of developing psychosis:

a) Are more likely to have an elevated BMI.
b) Are no more likely to smoke.
c) Eat diets higher in calories.
d) Are just as physically active.

5. Increased risk of developing diabetes:

a) Is associated with, but not caused by, antipsychotic medication.
b) Is not observed in families of people with severe mental illness.
c) Does not occur in healthy volunteers taking antipsychotics.
d) Can occasionally result in a life-threatening state following antipsychotic initiation that reverses on cessation of the antipsychotic responsible.

6. Which of the following did Myles et al. (2012) conclude about tobacco use in people with a first episode of psychosis:

a) 20% are regular smokers.
b) They are twice as likely to smoke than peers without psychosis.
c) Reduces anxiety.
d) Most individuals start smoking several years before the onset of psychosis.

7. Physical activity and sedentariness:

a) Sedentariness provides a self-regulatory mechanism for reducing co-existing stress in people experiencing psychosis.

b) People with psychosis are no more sedentary than peers without psychosis.
c) 60% of people with psychotic illnesses like schizophrenia are regularly active.
d) One extra hour of sedentary time increases the odds of developing type 2 diabetes and metabolic syndrome in the general population.

8. Which of the following factors might adversely effect the physical health of people with first-episode psychosis?

a) Socioeconomic disadvantage
b) Stigma and isolation
c) Side effects of anti-psychotic medication
d) All of the above

9. According to Stubbs et al. (2015), in people with established psychosis how much higher are rates of type 2 diabetes than in the general population?

a) 10 times
b) No different
c) 5–6 times
c) 2–3 times

10. According to Curtis et al. (2015), what % of service users gained more than 7% of initial baseline weight when standard care was supplemented with a 12-week individualised weight management intervention?

a) 13%
b) 30%
c) 75%
d) 30%

# INTRODUCTION

Healing is a matter of time but it is sometimes also a matter of opportunity. (Hippocrates 460–377 BC)

The idea that intervening earlier in the course of psychosis might improve downstream outcomes has underpinned significant advances in mental health practice in the last two decades:

I now believe that early intervention (in psychosis) will be the most important and far reaching reform of the National Service Framework (NSF) era … I think early intervention will have the greatest effect on people's lives. (Professor Louis Appleby, National Director for Mental Health, 10 October 2008, Personal communication)

Nevertheless, and notwithstanding the undoubted gains made by this National Institute for Health and Care Excellence-recommended service development

(NICE, 2013b: CG155, and 2014a: CG178), the current *scandal of premature mortality* remains largely unaddressed. In this chapter, we will argue that this early intervention reform is incomplete without the achievement of improved physical health outcomes.

We will highlight how people with serious mental illness have missed out on several decades of investment in prevention of cardiovascular disease and diabetes, and that these disorders are major contributors to a widening health gap. And yet, these disorders can be anticipated from adverse cardiometabolic risks that often accumulate early in the course of psychosis. Indeed, some risks can be directly attributed to the medications prescribed.

We will conclude by highlighting some encouraging new service innovations that attempt to address these risks much earlier. We will also describe a new international initiative entitled Healthy Active Lives (HeAL) which challenges the current lack of attention given to this health inequality. This UK-supported international consensus calls on health practitioners and service planners to reduce the likelihood of future life-shortening illness by paying much greater attention to cardiovascular and metabolic health in the critical early phase of psychosis and its treatment.

## THE EARLY PHASE OF PSYCHOSIS: A KEY TIME TO KEEP THE BODY IN MIND

Epidemiologist Geoffrey Rose, in a seminal paper (Rose, 1981), criticised the NHS for failing to address the problem of rising premature mortality from cardiovascular disease in the UK at that time. Rose called for an urgent strategic shift to a population-based prevention approach aimed at reversing the underlying faults rather than focusing purely on treating individual patients presenting with largely irreversible disease end-states like stroke and heart attack.

Nevertheless, for those experiencing serious mental illness, despite several decades of NHS investment in population-wide prevention initiatives, cardiovascular disease remains the most frequent cause of their premature death. This has occurred in the face of the evidence presented in Chapter 2, showing that potentially modifiable risk factors predictive of future cardiovascular disease and diabetes are more prevalent and arise from a younger age in people with mental health problems than for the general population. Indeed, the 15–20-year life-expectancy gap appears to be still widening, which suggests that this vulnerable population may still be missing out on benefits that the general population have steadily accrued through programmes such as the NICE-recommended NHS Health Check (NICE, 2014b: local government briefing (LGB)15) and incentivised schemes in primary care such as the Quality Outcome Framework (NHS Employers, 2016).

⚙ **REFLECTION POINT 6.1**

Think about how the NHS approaches cardiovascular risk reduction, perhaps reflecting on your own, or family, experiences. Then ask yourself why these approaches may be widening the mortality gap and increasing health inequalities experienced by people with serious mental illness.

Given the particular contributions of cardiovascular disease and diabetes to the poor health and reduced life expectancy of people with serious mental illness, Rose's hypothesis remains relevant to this vulnerable group and the challenge becomes one of targeting effective prevention measures before potentially modifiable risks for future disease become irreversibly entrenched.

To optimise the opportunities for prevention, we need particularly to examine those modifiable risks present in the early phase of psychosis that predict future cardiovascular disease and diabetes. These arise from a mixture of genetic and environmental influences. The latter are often linked with socioeconomic disadvantage and mediated through poor lifestyle choices and health risk behaviours, no different in essence from the general population. However, for those with mental illness, these influences may be further compounded by factors linked to the mental illness itself, adverse effects of psychiatric treatments and inequitable healthcare.

We have included genetic influence in this discussion because, although not modifiable, this should be taken into account when considering how individual vulnerability to specific risks may vary across a population with mental health problems. To illustrate this, consider the variation in incidence of major mental illness: while genetic variation explains some vulnerability, social deprivation may cause several-fold variation found between affluent and poor communities (Kirkbride et al., 2014). In a similar manner, genetic variation may influence individual vulnerability to heart disease and diabetes but socioeconomic gradients also account for variations in the likelihood of developing these conditions within the general population.

Notwithstanding the complexity of interactions between genes and environment, we need to consider body and mind together and holistically when thinking about ways to reduce these particular health inequalities. And the thesis of this chapter is that this integrated body and mind approach should commence as early as possible. The question is: *How early is early?*

Some health risk behaviours predate emergence of psychosis. A recent systematic review (Carney et al., 2016) observed those at high risk of developing psychosis to be more likely to smoke, to be less physically active and to have diets higher in calories, than peers not at high risk for psychosis. Cannabis use is another important health risk behaviour, not only increasing the likelihood of developing psychosis but of also stimulating appetite and higher calorie intake (Fergusson et al., 2006). Nevertheless, despite these differences in health risk behaviours, the body mass index appears to be no higher in those at high risk of psychosis compared with their peers (Carney et al., 2016).

However, that quickly changes with the onset of psychosis. A systematic review by Foley and Morley (2011) found significant weight gain and glucose and lipid disturbance developed within eight weeks of commencing antipsychotics, and continued to rise over the 12 months studied. Metabolic disturbances are common, affecting a third of individuals within 8 months of psychosis onset (Curtis et al., 2012).

Two studies of the relative prevalence of metabolic syndrome underline the magnitude and time frame of cardiometabolic risk acquisition. Prior to commencing antipsychotics, metabolic syndrome appears no more likely in people experiencing their first episode of psychosis, compared to peers without psychosis (Fleischhacker et al., 2013). However by age 40, people with schizophrenia were almost four times more likely to experience metabolic syndrome than age-matched peers without schizophrenia (Saari et al., 2005). Importantly, people with metabolic syndrome, compared to those without are (Alberti et al., 2005):

- Twice as likely to die from, and three times as likely to experience, a heart attack or stroke.
- Five times as likely to develop type 2 diabetes.

Thus, cardiometabolic risk establishes quickly with the emergence of psychosis and then steadily accumulates to pose an increasing threat to future health.

## KEY MESSAGE 6.1

In answering the question *'How early is early?'* we have shown that, in terms of cardiometabolic risk acquisition and the potential timing of opportunities for prevention:

- Significant health risk behaviours may be at play even prior to the onset of psychosis.
- Weight gain and metabolic disturbance become obvious with the onset of psychosis, often accelerating in the early treatment phase.
- Once commenced, a trajectory of accumulating cardiovascular and metabolic risk may continue, so that many individuals with serious mental illness by the age of 40 show a wide divergence in relative risk and are established on a path to premature cardiovascular disease and diabetes.

The implications for physical health and fitness of people at high risk of developing psychosis were reviewed in Chapter 5. But, for the remainder of this chapter, we will focus on those experiencing their first episode of psychosis.

# POTENTIALLY MODIFIABLE CARDIOMETABOLIC RISK: TARGETS FOR INTERVENTION FROM THE ONSET OF PSYCHOSIS AND ITS TREATMENT

---

### 👥 CASE STUDY 6.1

Jane is 30 years old and has been unwell for 12 months. She recently lost her job, lives in a high-rise flat and struggles to pay the rent. She complains that the medication makes her so drowsy and muddled that she can barely manage a conversation. She feels ashamed and shuns her family and friends, spending her day watching TV, smoking and snacking to relieve boredom and continual craving for food.

---

In order to understand why major metabolic disturbance should 'lift off' in the early treatment phase, it is important to appreciate the broader impact of developing psychosis. Beyond purely distress from symptoms, there may be profound social consequences with disrupted relationships, dashed aspirations for education and employment and fragile accommodation arrangements. Peak onset of psychosis in late teens and early adulthood (Kirkbride et al., 2006) coincides with rapid social, psychological and biological transition. Economic stability may be threatened, for instance employment rates plummet to 5–15% within a year (Killackey et al., 2006). These difficulties interweave with illness and treatment impacts to accentuate: unhealthy lifestyles; social issues such as perceived and actual stigma, isolation from friends, boredom, lack of finance to attend leisure activities; illness issues such as lack of motivation and paranoid thinking; and treatment issues such as sedation and poor concentration, and stimulation of appetite. It is hardly surprising that the end result is a measurable impact on:

- Poor diet – high in fat and refined sugar, low in dietary fibre and inadequate fruit and vegetable intake (Dipasquale et al., 2013).
- Physical inactivity – only 30% of people with psychotic illnesses like schizophrenia are regularly active, compared to 62% for non-psychiatric peers (Lindamer et al., 2008).
- Sedentariness – a recent systematic review by Stubbs et al. (2016) found that people with psychosis were sedentary for over 11 hours a day, and 3 hours more than their non-psychiatric peers. To put this in context, a study of the general population revealed that one extra hour of sedentary time was associated with 22% more type 2 diabetes and 39% more metabolic syndrome (van der Berg et al., 2016).

Add to these the impact of tobacco use (see Chapter 8 for more detail about smoking in people with mental health problems), the leading preventable cause of death in the UK. Emphasising its importance in early psychosis, a systematic review by Myles et al. (2012) found that 59% of those presenting with psychosis for the first time were already smoking. They were also six times more likely to smoke than their peers without psychosis, and the majority had started smoking several years before the onset of psychosis.

Thus, the early phase of psychosis constitutes a critical period of vulnerability, when health risk behaviours and wider social determinants come together with adversities created by the illness and its treatment.

---

### ⚙ REFLECTION POINT 6.2

Think about your clinical practice and how you approach the physical health of service users commencing treatment for psychosis:

- List the aspects of their health that you generally enquire about.
- What assessments do you make?
- What actions do you usually take to promote health?

---

## WEIGHT GAIN AND ANTIPSYCHOTIC MEDICATION

Antipsychotic treatment can cause people with psychosis to gain weight (see Chapter 9). Addington and colleagues (2006) observed that most weight gain occurred within the first three years of psychosis. The magnitude of early antipsychotic-induced weight gain was demonstrated by a systematic review – about 12 kg within the first 24 months, the rate slowing subsequently (Álvarez-Jiménez et al., 2008). The authors commented that most studies reviewed were of poor quality, short duration and chose subjects with established illness, many already having gained weight from previous antipsychotic exposure – and leading to a 3–4-fold underestimation of weight gain in those with first-episode psychosis. By contrast, the high-quality European First Episode Schizophrenia Trial (EUFEST) found that about 65% of people experiencing psychosis for the first time gained more than 7% of body weight during the first year of treatment (Kahn et al., 2008). This study and others like it confirm a causal link between antipsychotic medicines and weight gain, and also show how individual drugs vary in their propensity to cause weight gain (Tarricone et al., 2010; Foley and Morley, 2011).

What all these studies demonstrate is that weight gain can be rapid and substantial following antipsychotic initiation. Several factors can predict vulnerability to weight gain – these include: younger age, low BMI prior to starting treatment, concordant use of cannabis and non-white ethnicity (Holt and Peveler, 2009). Genetic variation in how individuals metabolise and respond to specific drugs may also contribute to differing susceptibilities to antipsychotic-induced weight gain (Zhang and Malhotra, 2011).

## METABOLIC DISTURBANCE

Weight gain, particularly when centrally distributed, may drive disturbances of glucose and lipid metabolism. Underlining how quickly metabolic disturbance can happen, the US RAISE study of 394 subjects with first-episode psychosis and an average age 23.6, observed significant dyslipidemia and impaired glucose handling after only 6–7 weeks' lifetime exposure to antipsychotics. The authors commented that the observed 56.3% prevalence of dyslipidemia was at least as common as the 53% prevalence observed in a general US population averaging 20 years older (Correll et al., 2014).

---

### 👤👤👤 CASE STUDY 6.2

It's ten weeks since Peter, aged 18, first presented with psychosis. You recall that he is a keen runner but notice that he appears pale and lethargic. You ask him whether he is enjoying his running and if the treatment is suiting. Peter responds, 'The last few weeks – no energy – can hardly get beyond my front door, let alone put on my trainers.' You arrange a random blood glucose estimation – 24 mmol/l. Peter has developed diabetes. You note that his weight is lower than when he first presented with psychosis.

---

Links between diabetes and psychosis are not a new observation, with Sir Henry Maudsley noting genetic susceptibility over a century ago: 'Diabetes is a disease which often shows itself in families in which insanity prevails' (Maudsley, 1879). Impaired glucose handling has been observed even prior to antipsychotic initiation (Ryan et al., 2003). However, a recent systematic review found little evidence of impaired glucose handling and metabolic syndrome in people with first-episode psychosis before commencing antipsychotic medication (Mitchell et al., 2013a). There is unequivocal evidence that antipsychotic medication can directly cause diabetes. In a double-blind study, healthy volunteers with neither mental illness nor obesity, when randomised to olanzapine or aripiprazole developed insulin resistance within nine days, compared with placebo (Teff et al., 2013). Moreover, antipsychotic-induced type 2 diabetes, although uncommon, has been observed in young people experiencing early psychosis. A recent systematic review of those under the age of 24 (average age of 14) found cumulative risk and exposure-adjusted incidences of type 2 diabetes were higher in antipsychotic-exposed youth than in healthy controls and psychiatric controls (Galling et al., 2016). And once psychosis becomes established, this population can expect two to three times more diabetes than the general population (Stubbs et al., 2015).

**KEY MESSAGE 6.2**

Cardiometabolic risk establishes in early psychosis:

- 59% of people with a first episode of psychosis are regular smokers.
- The majority gain more than 7% body weight within the first 12 months of treatment.
- Antipsychotic-induced weight gain and metabolic disturbance is detectable within weeks of initiating treatment.
- After 7 weeks of antipsychotic exposure, dyslipidemia rates in a US study of people with first-episode psychosis were at least as high as for the general population, 20 years older.

# FEEL MORE CONFIDENT IN SUPPORTING A PERSON EXPERIENCING PSYCHOSIS FOR THE FIRST TIME SO AS TO AVOID FUTURE POOR HEALTH FROM CARDIOVASCULAR DISEASE AND DIABETES

We want to conclude this chapter by considering how the early phase of psychosis may provide opportunities for developing and strengthening clinical practice to avoid downstream physical health problems such as cardiovascular disease and diabetes.

**CASE STUDY 6.3**

Shana, aged 24, attends for review. Her paranoid symptoms have diminished and she describes the voices as less threatening since commencing treatment for psychosis four weeks ago. Prior to this illness, she was slim and a keen swimmer. Despite improved psychiatric symptoms, she is upset, complaining: 'My weight has increased and my usual clothes no longer fit. Should I expect this?'

The case study above illustrates some dilemmas facing individuals and their practitioners, and why the early phase of psychosis presents an important opportunity to mitigate risks of future poor health. And, of course, risks to future health are not the only concerns. Severe weight gain may also threaten self-esteem and social participation, on top of having to adapt to emerging mental illness, increasing the sense of isolation and hopelessness. The impacts are reflected in a recent qualitative study by McCloughen and colleagues (2016) of young people affected by psychotic or mood disorders of severity sufficient to require admission and psychotropic medication. The participants confirmed how weight increase and limited exercise adversely impacted their lives and self-image, comparing this with their held belief for a holistic ideal of what constituted good physical health. And, yet, most participants simply accepted that their physical health would be compromised by medication side effects like sedation and increased appetite, without questioning the value of medications or discussing side effects and ways to mitigate them. Also demonstrated in this study, is how individuals can be unclear about what constitutes a legitimate reason to seek support for physical health – for instance, feeling that they had to be 'really sick' before they could approach their GP or dentist.

---

⚙️ **REFLECTION POINT 6.3**

Reflect on your experience of supporting service users newly diagnosed with psychosis and dealing with adverse effects of medication such as rapid weight gain. Aside from concerns for 'downstream' health problems like diabetes, what are the more immediate concerns that might trouble them?

---

Lack of clarity over clinical responsibility for physical health may extend to professionals in primary and secondary care and may partially explain the inadequate physical health monitoring observed in the National Audit of Schizophrenia (NAS) (Crawford et al., 2014). To address the poor performance identified, the NAS collaborated with the Royal Colleges of Psychiatrists, of General Practitioners and of Nursing, in order to adapt an original Australian resource for UK use, which was the Lester Positive Cardiometabolic Health Resource. This was updated in 2014 and endorsed by NICE, NHS England, Public Health England, Rethink and Diabetes UK (Shiers et al., 2014). Subsequently, Mental Health Trusts in England were incentivised to implement the Lester resource through a national Commissioning for Quality and Innovation Guidance (CQUIN) in 2015 which extended this to include early intervention in psychosis (EIP) services (NHS England, 2015b).

Recommendations on clinical responsibility in recent NICE guidance and standards (NICE, 2014a: CG178, 2013b: CG155, 2015: quality standard (QS)80) are particularly relevant to EIP:

- Secondary care teams should assess the service user's physical health and the effects of antipsychotic medication for at least the first 12 months or until the person's condition has stabilised, whichever is longer.
- Thereafter, assessments may be transferred to primary care under shared care arrangements and should take place at least annually.

## WHAT DO WE KNOW ABOUT PHYSICAL HEALTH MONITORING PERFORMANCE IN EARLY PSYCHOSIS?

The National Audit of Schizophrenia surveyed case records mainly from those with established schizophrenia, limiting understanding of what happened in Early Intervention for Psychosis services. However, the recent quality improvement programme run by Advancing Quality Alliance (AQuA) supporting five EIP services in Northern England gives some insights (Greenwood and Shiers, 2016). This improvement programme utilised a quality standard derived from the Lester resource, requiring services to demonstrate recorded screening for weight or BMI, smoking status, blood glucose, blood lipid and blood pressure, as well as positive family history of diabetes or premature cardiovascular disease. About 500 service users, aged 14–61, participated. The baseline audit revealed that fewer than 10% of cases received comprehensive screening, with rates rising to 60–80% across the five services at re-audit following AQuA's 6-month quality improvement programme (ibid.). While these improvements show the benefits of prioritising this issue, the baseline audit suggested that some EIP services' performance may be even poorer than that revealed by the NAS. Audits like the NAS and AQuA raise an ethical concern that vulnerable individuals are prescribed medication that can directly cause weight gain and metabolic disturbance, yet the monitoring for adverse effects is inadequate. This reinforces concerns raised by service users and carers about inadequate physical healthcare and prescribing practice as reported by the Schizophrenia Commission (2012) and backs up the Commission's call for the implementation of the Lester resource.

Responding to dissatisfactions of the sort described above, an international consensus has emerged, led by colleagues in Australia and the UK and now involving users, carers, clinicians and researchers from over 12 countries. Launched by the International Early Psychosis Association in November 2014, HeAL provides a *call to arms* for health practitioners and service providers to pay far greater attention to the cardiometabolic health of their service users in the critical early treatment phase of psychosis (Shiers and Curtis, 2014). HeAL advocates for patient-centred choice from the very first therapeutic encounter. This is entirely consistent with relevant NICE guidance, and includes access to individual and family psychological interventions, support for healthier lifestyles, and high-quality antipsychotic prescribing supported by collaborative treatment decisions that balance trade-offs between medication benefits and side effects.

HeAL sets out a number of measurable standards designed to raise expectations from those using services from the start of treatment, as illustrated in Reflection Point 6.4.

---

### ⚙ REFLECTION POINT 6.4

How might you support the HeAL objective that 75% of people with a first episode of psychosis gain no more than 7% of their pre-illness weight in the two years after initiating antipsychotic treatment? Think about at least one aspect of your clinical practice for each of these:

- Prescribing practice.
- Providing health checks.
- Offering health promotion.

## PRESCRIBING PRACTICE AND PROVIDING HEALTH CHECKS

People experiencing psychosis for the first time may be particularly sensitive to antipsychotic medication and require specific prescribing considerations – see the British Association of Psychopharmacologists' guidance (Barnes et al., 2011). They may be prone to early and sometimes rapid weight and metabolic disturbance, with olanzapine and clozapine being the most likely to cause this. These impacts can be greater in young patients and NICE has recently recommended that when considering prescribing antipsychotics for adolescents and children, they should be advised that olanzapine is more likely to cause greater weight gain than other second-generation antipsychotics and that this can develop quickly.

The Lester resource reflects NICE guidance in recommending a schedule of physical health monitoring that can alert practitioners to early weight gain and metabolic disturbances (Table 6.1). This is important because early rapid weight gain (for example, 5% weight gain in the first month) predicts those more likely to develop severe weight gain in the longer term (Vandenberghe et al., 2015) and similarly for metabolic disturbance. This should prompt an urgent treatment review to consider switching antipsychotic medication and intensifying lifestyle interventions. Occasionally, glucose and lipid disturbance occurs rapidly without weight gain – the need for clinical vigilance emphasised by reports of rare but potentially life-threatening diabetes that may reverse on withdrawing the antipsychotic responsible (McIntyre et al., 2001).

**Table 6.1   Schedule for physical health monitoring in people newly prescribed antipsychotic medication**

| Monitoring schedule | Initial baseline | Weekly for first 6 weeks | At 12 weeks | Then annually |
|---|---|---|---|---|
| Family history of diabetes or premature CVD | X | | | X |
| Lifestyle review – smoking, diet and physical activity | X | | X | X |
| Weight (BMI and/or waist circumference) | X | X | X | X |
| Blood pressure | X | | X | X |
| Glucose (fasting blood glucose or $HbA_{1C}$)[1] | X | | X | X |
| Lipid profile[1] | X | | X | X |

*Note*:

[1] If fasting samples cannot be obtained, a non-fasting sample is satisfactory.

Finally, there is currently interest in a number of adjunctive pharmacological approaches to mitigate antipsychotic-induced weight gain – Metformin shows the most consistent benefits but studies to date have been few and of short duration. Most authorities advise that primary lifestyle approaches should be the first option (Manu et al., 2015).

---

### KEY MESSAGE 6.3

When prescribing antipsychotics to people experiencing psychosis for the first time:

- Base antipsychotic choice on an individual's relative liability to side effects.
- Consider individual service user preference.
- Provide low-dose initiation and titration of dosage within British National Formulary range.
- Ensure systematic monitoring of side effects from the start of treatment.

For detailed prescribing considerations for first-episode psychosis, see the British Association of Psychopharmacologists' guidance (Barnes et al., 2011).

---

## OFFERING HEALTH PROMOTION

Notwithstanding evidence that prevention approaches such as weight-reducing programmes can be effective (Bartels, 2015), these interventions have generally targeted individuals with established psychosis. HeAL challenges services to provide these interventions much earlier when risk factors may be more amenable to alteration. It is worth noting that avoidance/mitigation of weight gain is the objective here, rather than necessarily weight reduction, because, typically, over 65% of individuals experiencing a first episode of psychosis gain more than 7% of initial baseline weight within 12 months (Kahn et al., 2008), beginning to accrue within weeks of commencing treatment. Weight management programmes to supplement usual care have recently been evaluated in some 'real-world' Early Intervention for Psychosis service settings.

---

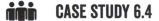 **CASE STUDY 6.4**

Curtis and colleagues (2015) prospectively compared two EIP services in New South Wales, one service acting as a 'standard care' control to the other service, in which standard care was supplemented by a 12-week individualised programme of weight management consisting of health coaching, dietetic support and a supervised exercise programme. Of those receiving 'standard care', 75% gained significant weight (>7% of initial baseline weight), compared to only 13% in the intervention group.

---

**CASE STUDY 6.5**

In the UK, Smith and colleagues (2015) supplemented Worcestershire's EIP service with access to a weight management programme delivered through partnership with the Health and Wellbeing programme of Worcestershire University. With similarities to the New South Wales intervention group (Curtis et al., 2015), a 12-week programme included health coaching, individualised nutrition advice and group exercise programme. About a quarter of those eligible took up the programme, with benefits in terms of avoiding weight gain equivalent to the New South Wales intervention group (Smith et al., 2015).

---

Both of these service case studies demonstrate practice-based evidence for a multimodal approach that not only provides systematic monitoring for adverse changes, but also guarantees high-quality prescribing while supporting service users to make healthier lifestyle choices. They reflect the '*Don't just screen, intervene*' mantra of the Lester resource through an optimistic approach and raised expectation from those who both use and provide these services. These encouraging service developments coincide with Achieving Better Access, a major policy initiative in England to further strengthen EIP services (NHS England, 2015a).

## CONCLUSION

Healing is a matter of time but it is sometimes also a matter of opportunity. (Hippocrates 460–377 BC)

We have argued in this chapter for a radical shift in the nature and focus of interventions to counter the build-up of cardiometabolic risk for individuals in the critical early phase of psychosis and its treatment. An aggressive trajectory of increasing cardiometabolic disturbance places many of this population at significant risk in their twenties and thirties, at an age before routine cardiovascular disease prevention is usually considered. Furthermore, despite some encouraging evidence that prevention approaches such as smoking cessation and weight-reducing programmes can be effective, these interventions have generally been targeted at individuals with established psychosis when risk factors may be less amenable to alteration. The ongoing Early Intervention for Psychosis reform has a real opportunity to ensure that the *scandal of premature mortality* is tackled from the start of psychosis and its treatment. Much of what is needed to prevent these risks accruing does not require new technology or sophisticated training – many simple measures could be introduced into routine care immediately. By applying a holistic *body and mind* approach right from the first clinical encounter, obesity, diabetes and premature death from cardiovascular disease need not and, indeed, should not, be inevitable consequences of psychosis and its treatment.

## USEFUL RESOURCES

British Association for Psychopharmacology. Available at: www.bap.org.uk/guidelines (accessed 5 August 2016).

This provides:

- Evidence-based guidelines for the pharmacological treatment of schizophrenia: recommendations from the British Association for Psychopharmacology, 2011.
- Guidelines on the management of weight gain, metabolic disturbances and cardiovascular risk associated with psychosis and antipsychotic drug treatment, 2016.

Healthy Active Lives (HeAL) (2013) Consensus Statement, 2013, iphYs (International Physical Health in Youth) special interest group. Available at: www.iphys.org.au (accessed 5 August 2016).

Lester UK Adaptation (2014) *Positive Cardiometabolic Health* Resource, update. Available at: www.rcpsych.ac.uk/quality/NAS/resources (accessed 5 August 2016).

## ANSWERS TO MULTIPLE CHOICE QUESTIONS

1(a), 2(c), 3(d), 4(c), 5(d), 6(d), 7(d), 8(d), 9(d), 10(a)

# SEVEN

## PROMOTING PHYSICAL ACTIVITY

### JOSEPH FIRTH AND REBEKAH CARNEY

## CHAPTER LEARNING OUTCOMES

After reading this chapter, you will be able to:

- Describe the relationship between physical activity and wellbeing.
- Understand how physical inactivity and poor fitness impacts on physical health and functional recovery in people with mental health problems.
- Analyse barriers to increasing physical activity in people with mental health problems and consider how they may be overcome.
- Examine evidence-supported approaches to increasing physical activity and their benefits to wellbeing.

## MULTIPLE CHOICE QUESTIONS

We have included 10 multiple choice questions at the beginning of this chapter for readers wishing to test their knowledge of its contents. We have included the answers at the end of the chapter, but advise you not to check these until you have answered them before and after reading the chapter so that you can determine how much your knowledge has increased.

1. Taking up regular physical activity and exercise reduces people's risk of:

   a) Cancer.
   b) Premature mortality.
   c) Heart disease.
   d) All of the above.

2. The NHS guidelines on exercise in the UK recommends that all adults achieve:

   a) 150 minutes of moderate activity per week.
   b) 75 minutes of vigorous activity per week.
   c) 90–100 minutes of moderate-to-vigorous activity per week.
   d) Any of the above.

*(Continued)*

*(Continued)*

3. Low-intensity exercise, such as household chores or steady walking:

   a) Is no different to sitting on the sofa.
   b) Is just enough to stay in top health if you do it often.
   c) Fails to improve physical health to the same extent as moderate-to-vigorous exercise.
   d) Should always be the main goal for any physical health intervention.

4. People with severe mental illness are:

   a) More sedentary than the general population.
   b) Less likely to exercise than the general population.
   c) Both more sedentary and less likely to exercise than the general population.
   d) More physically active than the general population.

5. Exercise interventions should be implemented as early as possible after the onset of mental illness because:

   a) Clinical trials have proven that exercise is more effective for improving mental health in younger service users.
   b) Only young people will ever get involved with exercise training.
   c) The early stages are a crucial period for preventing weight gain, metabolic dysfunction and functional disability before they arise.
   d) People with long-term conditions will not benefit from exercise.

6. Nyboe et al. (2015) recently found that, for people commencing antipsychotic treatment, the most accurate predictor of their 1-year health outcomes is their:

   a) Fitness.
   b) Physical activity levels.
   c) Eating habits.
   d) BMI.

7. Trials of exercise for people with schizophrenia have found that increases in fitness correlate with reductions in:

   a) Positive symptoms (hallucinations and delusions).
   b) Negative symptoms (low motivation and blunted affect).
   c) Cognitive symptoms (memory and processing speed deficits).
   d) Functional disability.

8. Which of the following approaches has been found to be ineffective for increasing physical activity in people with severe mental illness:

   a) Building exercise facilities into mental health clinics and services.
   b) Supporting people to engage with exercise available through their local communities.
   c) Providing people with standardised advice and information on how much exercise they should do.
   d) Using fitness 'apps' to encourage people to exercise at home.

9. The most common motivations for physical activity expressed by service users include:

   a) Fitness and weight loss.
   b) Social aspects and meeting new friends.
   c) Enjoyment of exercise.
   d) Preventing boredom.

10. Ultimately, the best type of activity to get people who are new to exercise to engage in is:

    a) Aerobic training, such as cycling and running.
    b) Strength exercises and weight training.
    c) Sports and group fitness classes.
    d) The type of exercise that they personally feel most motivated to do.

# INTRODUCTION

This chapter will consider how the reduced levels of physical activity observed in people with mental health problems may contribute to their poor physical health status. Following this, the physical and psychological benefits of physical activity interventions for this population will be outlined, and the evidence for determining optimal amounts/types of exercise will be reviewed. The chapter will conclude by reviewing the common barriers towards physical activity among people with mental health problems and then describing how these can be effectively overcome using empirically based strategies that have been proven to be effective in a recent clinical trial.

# RELATIONSHIPS BETWEEN EXERCISE AND WELLBEING

## PHYSICAL ACTIVITY AND POPULATION HEALTH

The World Health Organization (2009) recently placed 'physical inactivity' as the fourth largest cause of mortality worldwide. Physical inactivity is also strongly associated with three of the other top five mortality causes, with high blood pressure placing first, high blood glucose third and obesity fifth. Additionally, a recent large-scale European study found that inactivity is responsible for twice as many deaths as obesity each year (Ekelund et al., 2015). Along with premature mortality, physical inactivity also increases the risk of long-term conditions such as diabetes, heart disease and breast cancer (Lee et al., 2012). In the UK, physical inactivity is considered one of the greatest public health issues (Blair, 2009).

    The promotion of physical activity can be separated into two aims. The first is decreasing the amount of 'sedentary behaviour', which generally refers to sitting time (but not sleeping). The second is increasing the amount of time spent 'exercising', defined as: 'any structured and repetitive physical activity for improving/maintaining physical fitness' (Caspersen et al., 1985). To maintain good physical health, the UK NHS guidelines recommend that all adults achieve at least 150 minutes of 'moderate' exercise, or 75 minutes of 'vigorous' exercise, each week, along with muscle-strengthening activities (Department of Health, 2011). Alternatively, a mixture of the two intensities (for example, 90–100 minutes of moderate-to-vigorous activity) can fulfil the recommendations.

# WHAT CONSTITUTES 'MODERATE' OR 'VIGOROUS' ACTIVITY?

Generally, no specific activities are strictly categorised as moderate or vigorous, as the intensity of exercise for any individual lies in relation to their own fitness levels. While jogging or football may constitute 'moderate' exercise for an active 18-year-old, these same activities would be 'vigorous' exercise for an overweight, inactive 45-year-old. NHS guidelines define moderate exercise as: 'activity which noticeably increases the heart rate, breathing, and body temperature, while still leaving one feeling able to talk'. Vigorous exercise 'results in hard breathing and rapid heart rate, leaving one unable to talk without stopping for breath'. The term 'low-intensity activity' can also be used when referring to casual walking or completing household chores. This is preferable to sedentary behaviour, but does not confer the same health benefits of moderate or vigorous exercise (Chastin et al., 2015). Only a third of UK adults meet the recommended amounts of exercise – making this the third most sedentary population in Europe.

> ⚙ **REFLECTION POINT 7.1**
>
> • For you, what would constitute 'moderate exercise' and what would count as 'vigorous exercise'? Which would you like to do more of?
> • Consider what would count as 'moderate' or 'vigorous' exercise for different people you know, including friends, family members and service users.

## *PHYSICAL ACTIVITY AND FITNESS LEVELS IN PEOPLE WITH MENTAL HEALTH PROBLEMS*

Unfortunately, physical activity is even lower among people with mental health problems. A recent meta-analysis showed that people with schizophrenia engaged in significantly less structured exercise and also greater amounts of sedentary behaviour than matched controls (Soundy et al., 2013). Additionally, people with mental health problems have significantly lower fitness levels than matched controls (Vancampfort et al., 2015b).

This inactivity and poor fitness is associated with a range of adverse health outcomes. For instance, Vancampfort et al. (2012) found that people with serious mental illness who sat for 10+ hours per day were more likely to be overweight and suffer from metabolic syndrome than those who sat for 5 hours per day. Similarly, service users who do not engage in regular moderate-to-vigorous exercise have worse cardiorespiratory health and higher risk of diabetes (ibid.).

These physical health problems also cause functional limitations and impact on service users' quality of life (Strassnig et al., 2012). Furthermore, inactivity and poor fitness are even associated with more negative symptoms (such as low motivation and anhedonia) and cognitive deficits (Kimhy et al., 2014; Vancampfort et al., 2015a). These symptoms are particularly detrimental to functional recovery (in Chapter 11, we describe an intervention called 'behavioural activation', developed specifically to help people with negative symptoms to increase their activity levels). Therefore, there is a clear need to increase physical activity in people with mental health problems.

---

### KEY MESSAGE 7.1

Inactivity is extremely damaging for physical health. People with mental health problems are less active than other members of the general population. The downsides of this include:

- Immediate weight gain from the onset of antipsychotic treatment.
- Long-term physical health conditions such as diabetes and heart disease.
- Functional disability and poor quality of life.

---

## PHYSICAL ACTIVITY OVER THE COURSE OF SERIOUS MENTAL ILLNESS

There is currently insufficient longitudinal research on physical activity in people with mental health problems to establish when sedentary habits arise. Nonetheless, a survey by Morgan et al. (2014) of over 1000 people with psychosis in Australia found that younger service users (aged 18–34) were significantly more active than the older service users (aged 35–65). Similarly, Walther et al. (2014) used wrist actigraphy to objectively measure physical activity in 149 people with psychosis, and found that those with first-episode psychosis were significantly more active than those with multi-episode psychosis, even when controlling for age, antipsychotic usage and negative symptoms. This suggests that physical activity decreases over the course of psychotic illness, independently of other factors.

---

### ⚙ REFLECTION POINT 7.2

- Which service users whom you know would be most easily engaged in some type of exercise?
- Write down three things that may impact on someone's ability to take up regular exercise. How could these be overcome or avoided?

# INCREASING PHYSICAL ACTIVITY: BENEFITS AND BARRIERS FOR PEOPLE WITH MENTAL HEALTH PROBLEMS

## *INCREASING PHYSICAL ACTIVITY TO REDUCE METABOLIC RISK*

Antipsychotics, although effective for reducing psychotic symptoms, are linked with severe metabolic side effects (De Hert et al., 2012). Rapid weight gain is common in the first year of treatment and the risk of metabolic syndrome increases fivefold (ibid., 2006). This, in turn, reduces self-esteem and increases feelings of stigma and discrimination (Barber et al., 2011). Furthermore, preventing cardiometabolic disorders is substantially more feasible and effective than attempting to reverse the long-term consequences (in Chapter 6, we emphasise the importance of timely interventions to prevent weight gain). Thus, the initial prescription of antipsychotics is the optimal period for increasing physical activity, when service users are more active, more readily engaged with exercise, and before metabolic disorders and obesity arise.

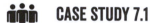 **CASE STUDY 7.1**

When he was 19 years old, Ahmed experienced his first episode of psychosis, resulting in him being prescribed antipsychotic medication. Before this, he had always been a slim-built young man, with no body issues whatsoever. By the time he was 21, Ahmed had gained 13 kg. This made him feel extremely self-conscious, resulting in social avoidance and severe bouts of depression. He has now started exercising to try and lose some weight, but told his personal trainer on multiple occasions how he wishes he had been more aware that he was likely to gain weight early on as he could have tried harder to prevent it.

Many variables affect the long-term health outcome of antipsychotic treatment. However, physical fitness is particularly protective against the metabolic side effects of treatment. A recent study conducted by Nyboe et al. (2015) examined the metabolic status (blood pressure, BMI and waist circumference) and health behaviours (physical activity, eating habits and smoking) of 99 people in their first year of antipsychotic treatment. Results showed that the only independent predictor of metabolic syndrome after a 1-year follow-up was aerobic fitness. Furthermore, aerobic fitness was one of the strongest predictors of each individual metabolic risk factor, such as waist circumference. Increases in aerobic fitness occur more rapidly than weight-loss exercise, and confer greater benefits for long-term health (Vancampfort et al., 2015b). Thus, physical health interventions for people with psychosis should specifically aim to improve this crucial variable.

## USING EXERCISE TO IMPROVE MENTAL HEALTH OUTCOMES

A recent meta-analysis of randomised controlled trials of exercise for people with schizophrenia (Firth et al., 2015) revealed that interventions which administer ≥90 minutes of moderate or vigorous exercise per week significantly reduced psychiatric symptoms. The benefits of exercise also appeared to be more dependent on the amount/intensity of activity achieved, rather than the type of exercise. Many different activities improved mental health (including cycling, fitness circuits and team sports), although interventions that used only low-intensity activity such as casual walking and stretching had no significant benefits.

Furthermore, negative symptoms and cognitive deficits were significantly reduced by moderate-to-vigorous exercise. This is particularly important, since these aspects of illness are very influential in long-term recovery, yet often left untreated (Arango et al., 2013). Again, first-episode psychosis may be an optimal period for exercise to improve mental health, since interventions that target negative symptoms early on can maximise functional recovery (Álvarez-Jiménez et al., 2012). Indeed, longitudinal studies have already shown that physical activity in early stages of illness is associated with better functional outcomes (Lee et al., 2013).

---

### KEY MESSAGE 7.2

The sooner we can offer exercise to service users, the better. This is because, in the early stages of illness, people are:

- Relatively free of cardiometabolic comorbidity.
- More able to engage with moderate/vigorous activities.
- Most likely to experience maximum psychosocial benefits from exercise.

---

## BARRIERS TO INCREASING EXERCISE IN PEOPLE WITH MENTAL HEALTH PROBLEMS

Unfortunately, simply providing access to leisure facilities and generic advice is entirely ineffective for increasing physical activity. For instance, Archie et al. (2003) offered people with a diagnosis of schizophrenia free gym memberships, with introductory sessions, but 90% of the participants stopped attending completely within less than 6 months. This poor engagement with exercise can also prevent service users from benefiting from the interventions. For example, in the TOPFIT study (Scheewe et al., 2013), significant improvements in mental health only occurred for the minority of participants who attended at least 50% of exercise sessions.

However, the majority of people with serious mental illness regard exercise as beneficial and enjoyable, and would like to use it to improve their physical health

(Bradshaw et al., 2012; Faulkner et al., 2007). Thus, it appears that an array of barriers actually prevent this population from engaging in exercise. To examine this, our research group conducted another meta-analysis of 12 independent studies examining the barriers to exercise expressed by 6431 service users (Firth et al., 2016c). The percentage of service users who reported each barrier is displayed in Figure 7.1. The most common barrier was 'low mood and stress' (experienced by 61% of service users). The second most common barrier was a 'lack of support' for exercise.

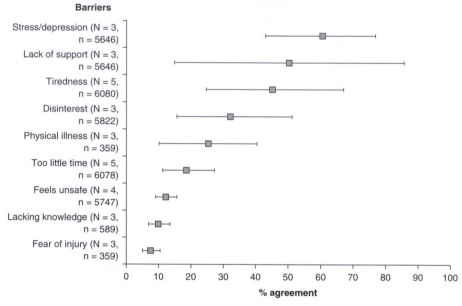

**Figure 7.1   Proportional meta-analyses of barriers to exercise in serious mental illness**

*Note*: The forest plot shows the percentage of service users experiencing each barrier (Box points) and the 95% CI (horizontal lines).

### ⚙ REFLECTION POINT 7.3

- Look at Figure 7.1. Is the ranking of any of these barriers surprising to you?
- Can you think of any that are missing but often present for people whom you work with?

## *MOTIVATIONS FOR INCREASING EXERCISE IN PEOPLE WITH MENTAL HEALTH PROBLEMS*

We also analysed the motivating factors for exercise in people with serious mental illness (Figure 7.2). 'Improving general health' was the most common reason for exercising, endorsed by 91% of participants. In the physical health categories, exercising to 'lose weight' was most popular (83%). This is unsurprising, given the high

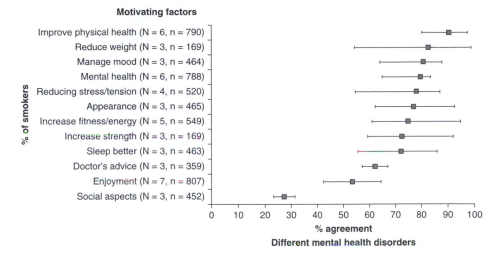

**Figure 7.2   Proportional meta-analyses of motivating factors for exercise in serious mental illness**

*Note*: The forest plot shows the percentage of participants agreeing with each motivating factor (Box points) and the 95% CI (horizontal lines).

rates of obesity and weight gain among people with serious mental illness (Vancampfort et al., 2015d). However, physical activity makes only a modest contribution to weight loss (Haskell et al., 2007), so dietary advice may also be required to achieve these goals.

Nonetheless, service users also acknowledged the psychological benefits of exercise, especially for 'improving mood' (81%) and 'reducing stress' (78%). Additionally, 'improving fitness' was a highly desirable benefit, expressed by 75% of participants. This is encouraging, since fitness is readily improved by exercise, and may be a key driver of the physical and mental benefits (Vancampfort et al., 2015b). Therefore, fitness outcomes should be emphasised when developing health interventions.

## KEY MESSAGE 7.3

Many people with serious illness would like to exercise more, but struggle to do so. Understanding the motivations and barriers in this population can help us to maximise exercise participation:

- The key psychological benefits of exercise recognised by service users (mood enhancement and stress reduction) are directly related to the barriers they experience towards it.
- Providing enough support to overcome these barriers could help people to achieve their exercise goals and engage in long-term physical activity.

# INDIVIDUALISED EXERCISE ROUTINES: FEASIBLE, EFFECTIVE AND MOTIVATING FOR SERVICE USERS

## *INDIVIDUALISED EXERCISE IN THE INVESTIGATING THE BENEFITS OF EXERCISE IN EARLY PSYCHOSIS (iBEEP) TRIAL*

*Note*: Links to all the free resources mentioned in this section are listed at the end of the chapter.

Various research groups have produced recommendations for administering exercise treatments for people with serious mental illness (Morgan et al., 2013; Rosenbaum et al., 2015). Collectively, these highlight the importance of implementing individualised exercise, and provide participants with autonomy to choose motivating types of exercise while also considering their personal incentives and barriers. Thus, the Investigating the Benefits of Exercise in Early Psychosis trial (iBEEP) was recently conducted by our research group in order to look into the feasibility of individualised exercise as an intervention for early psychosis (Firth et al., 2016a).

---

### ⚙ REFLECTION POINT 7.4

- Which athletes are the healthiest: Swimmers? Gymnasts? Rowers? They are all in great condition – even though they do totally different training. This reminds us that it is more important to encourage people towards exercise that they will actually enjoy and maintain, rather than trying to force them towards 'the best kind'.
- Write down a few activities which you think would be acceptable for people you know. What are the most common sorts of exercise that people do?

---

Participants for iBEEP were all receiving treatment for first-episode psychosis from the Early Intervention Services in Manchester in the UK. To deliver individualised exercise, we firstly designed personalised training programs for each participant. These aimed to achieve at least 90 minutes per week of moderate-to-vigorous activity, for 10 weeks, using any type of exercise they preferred. Routines were planned by research assistants who completed an 'exercise formulation questionnaire' (available online) with each participant, at the beginning of their programme.

Following this, research assistants arranged the participants' access to leisure services in their local community. 'Community leisure services' are now widespread in the UK, and offer subsidised fitness activities and gym memberships for anyone referred by the National Health Service (NHS). Research assistants were also offered to act as a 'training partner', and accompanied participants for up to two 1-hour sessions per week during their 10-week intervention. Attendance was recorded in an exercise logbook, which was completed on a weekly basis to detail the duration, modality and intensity of each exercise session.

This individualised approach proved successful: 93% of the 28 participants who commenced the intervention were retained over 10 weeks. Furthermore, the majority of participants actually exceeded their 90 minutes per week target, with participants achieving an average of 107 minutes of moderate-to-vigorous exercise each week. We also measured the participants' physical and mental health before-and-after the exercise intervention. Figure 7.3 displays changes in psychiatric symptoms in the exercise group as measured by the Positive and Negative Syndrome Scale (PANSS) (Kay et al., 1989), compared to a small group of matched participants from the same Early Intervention Services who were not receiving any exercise. Whereas the control group only had a 8% reduction of symptoms over 10 weeks (as might be expected from continued usual treatment), the exercise group had a 27% decrease in overall symptom scores (p = 0.001), which was statistically and clinically significant (Firth et al., 2016a).

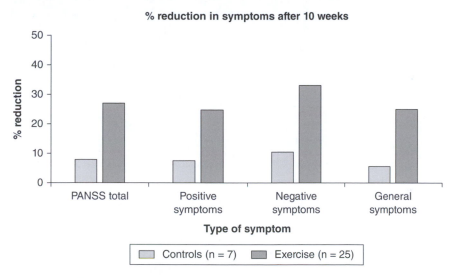

**Figure 7.3 iBEEP study outcomes**

*Note*: Bars show percentage reduction in psychiatric symptoms after 10 weeks. Darker colour represents those receiving the exercise intervention. Blue represents those receiving usual care.

Additionally, the exercise programme appeared to be effective for improving the physical health of service users: over the 10-week study, participants actually lost a small amount of weight (1 kg), thus avoiding the steep trajectory of weight gain typically observed in early psychosis. Furthermore, there was a significant reduction in waist circumference after the intervention (–2 cm, p = 0.008) and increased performance on a speed-walking fitness test, which almost reached statistical significance (p = 0.057). Given the short time frame of the study, these improvements indicate that, if participants could maintain their exercise over time, this could be one potential method for combating the metabolic side effects and weight gain associated with antipsychotic treatment.

Qualitative interviews were also used to explore participants' own experience of exercise (Firth et al., 2016b). Some key quotes are displayed in Key Message 7.4. These describe how engaging with exercise can inhibit hallucinations and intrusive thoughts, helping people to 'reconnect with reality' by focusing on physical exertion. This was also found to have an enduring impact on the rest of the person's day, reducing the usual feelings of disturbance or despair.

## KEY MESSAGE 7.4     SERVICE USER FEEDBACK

After analysing all the interviews with iBEEP's participants, some common themes emerged:

- Alleviating symptoms: 'When I'm training, the voices are suppressed, 'cos I'm so concentrated on lifting that weight up, doing the next exercise, that everything else clears out of your head.'
- Energising motivation: 'It makes me more active, before I was lazy and couldn't be bothered doing things. But, now, it's like I'm more active and I just want to go out there and start going to the gym … Got my get up and go back!'
- Boosting confidence: 'It makes me feel more happy in myself, you know, more confident, more self-esteem, you know, believe in myself better, a lot more.'

More qualitative feedback is available online (Firth et al., 2016b).

Qualitative quotes from participants also explained how exercise is an energising and uplifting activity, which helps people to overcome feelings of low energy and poor motivation. The greatest quantitative reductions from exercise were also observed in negative symptoms (Figure 7.3). These effects may be due to neurobiological responses to exercise, as participants reported a 'feel good' effect immediately after their sessions. The iBEEP study also assessed participants' neurocognitive functioning using computerised tests, both before and after the intervention, and found that exercise was associated with improved verbal memory and increased processing speed.

Therefore, exercise may offer an empowering and natural method for treating both negative and cognitive symptoms in early psychosis, which are mostly unresponsive to antipsychotic medication, but particularly important for functional recovery (Álvarez-Jiménez et al., 2012; Arango et al., 2013). These immediate benefits further indicate that exercise in early psychosis could improve long-term outcomes, as early intervention for negative symptoms and cognitive functioning may prevent enduring functional disability (Álvarez-Jiménez et al., 2012;

Bowie et al., 2014). Indeed, even after our relatively short intervention, significant improvements were observed in participants' social functioning (Firth et al., 2016a).

---

### KEY MESSAGE 7.5

The iBEEP study found that people with early psychosis engaged well with individualised exercise training. This resulted in:

- People achieving sufficient amounts of weekly exercise.
- Significant improvements in psychiatric symptoms and cognitive functioning.
- Participants themselves describing a wide range of benefits for their psychological wellbeing.

---

A further example of the effectiveness of individualised gym training is the 'In-Shape' trial (Bartels et al., 2013). In this study, 133 participants with long-term mental health problems were randomly assigned either to: (i) Control Group: gym membership plus fitness education; or (ii) In-Shape group: gym membership plus personalised fitness training. Results showed that the In-Shape group attended the gym three times more than the control condition. Furthermore, 50% of the In-Shape group significantly reduced their cardio-metabolic risk after 12 months. The iBEEP and In-Shape studies show us that individualised exercise programmes can overcome the sedentary lifestyles typically observed in people with serious mental illness, which has multiple benefits for physical and mental health.

---

### KEY MESSAGE 7.6    SERVICE USER FEEDBACK

Quotes from the iBEEP study show us which parts of the individualised interventions people value most:

- Choice: 'It's very important in drawing the individual towards making their own choice. They can make a choice in what they want to do, and what they love to do, it motivates them to sort of do what they feel happy to do.'
- Supporting autonomy: 'You've got someone there also who's basically saying, "It's alright I'm here. I'll show you what you need to learn" and once like the 6 months is over they've got that extra bit of confidence to say I'll give it a go on me own.'
- Overcoming barriers: 'If you can learn and do things in the gym, then you can do it anywhere outside and, you know, you can get other people involved as well … it definitely improves your lifestyle.'

## *PLANNING AND STARTING A NEW ROUTINE*

For the iBEEP study, we developed an 'Exercise Formulation Questionnaire' (available online) as a systematised method of planning individualised routines for service users. The central aspect of this questionnaire is a list of potential exercise activities, to be ranked in order of preference by participants. The questionnaire also explores participants' desired outcomes of exercise. Talking about people's incentives for exercise before commencing the routine naturally creates self-set goals, thus encouraging behavioural change (Dishman et al., 2009). This process also ensures that selected activities are appropriate for people's goals. For instance, the ideal activities for a service user who is hoping to gain muscle and improve body shape would differ substantially from someone looking to join a sports group for socialising and enjoyment. Finally, the questionnaire briefly assesses barriers towards exercise by asking participants what they would require to attend exercise sessions, since previous studies have identified 'lack of support' as a critical modifiable barrier towards exercise (Firth et al., 2016c). Therefore, iBEEP offered every participant accompaniment to exercise (from a research assistant), and helped plan transport to exercise facilities if required.

───────────── **ACTIVITY 7.1    PLANNING EXERCISE** ─────────────

The Exercise Formulation Questionnaires were used to create personalised exercise plans, designed to achieve at least 90 minutes of moderate-to-vigorous exercise per week, since this amount of exercise can improve mental health in psychotic disorders (ibid.):

- Print off one of the exercise questionnaires, and complete this as a practice. Now use this information to plan an exercise training programme for yourself!
- Consider whether the programme that you have planned would be feasible, readily available, affordable? And does it meet the 90-minutes-per-week recommendations?

## *ENGAGING PEOPLE IN INDIVIDUALISED EXERCISE*

Gym training was selected as a preferred type of exercise by all participants in the iBEEP study, even though they were offered many alternative activities (Table 7.1). Recent research indicates that combining aerobic with resistance exercise may be the optimal method for rapidly improving body composition, cardiometabolic risk and brain health (Church et al., 2010; Nouchi et al., 2014). For our study, a standardised iBEEP Exercise Guide (available online) was developed, with two different 'training sessions'. Each session aims for 45–60 minutes of moderate-to-vigorous aerobic activity and resistance exercises. The specific exercises used can be altered to participant preference. Options for aerobic-based exercise include treadmills,

**Table 7.1 Popularity of different exercise options in the iBEEP Study**

| Exercise type | Service users taking part n (%) | % of all exercise sessions recorded |
|---|---|---|
| Gym sessions: Supervised | 27 (96%) | 65.5 |
| Gym sessions: Alone | 14 (50%) | 13.3 |
| Football | 2 (11%) | 9 |
| Boxing/Martial Arts | 3 (11%) | 5 |
| Cycling | 2 (7%) | 4 |
| Badminton | 3 (7%) | 3 |
| Swimming | 3 (11%) | 2 |
| Gym: Fitness Classes | 3 (11%) | >1 |

*Source*: Firth et al. (2016d)

cycle ergometers, cross-trainers and rowing machines. Resistance training should prioritise exercises for the major muscle groups of legs, back and chest, before moving onto small muscles, such as the arms and abdominals.

The research assistants who accompanied participants had several years of gymnasium experience, but no formal qualifications in personal training/coaching. However, professional instruction was available from the qualified staff at community leisure centres, who conduct gym inductions and are able to provide further advice to all gym members, as required. Thus, such interventions can be delivered by any support staff who are enthusiastic about exercise. Embedding exercise within community services also received very positive feedback from service users, who found this to be beneficial for social integration and confidence. Although individualised programmes seem resource-intensive, they can usually be delivered in groups of 2–3 service users (as most prefer the same types of exercise). Furthermore, group-based exercise interventions also have higher retention rates and better adherence than solitary exercise (Firth et al., 2015; Vancampfort et al., 2015c).

As an alternative approach, setting up fitness rooms within mental health clinics can also be effective (Adams et al., 2015; Curtis et al., 2014). However, it should also be considered that mental health appointments are generally too infrequent to meet target amounts of weekly exercise. Instead, delivering exercise interventions through community leisure services confers several benefits. First, it is affordable, since community-based exercise can take advantage of existing facilities, readily available expertise and discounted memberships for NHS referred patients. Second, it encourages regular, sustainable exercise (independent of ongoing treatment). Third, it is naturally reintegrative, destigmatising and fosters an attitude of self-management of one's own health. Most drawbacks of community-based interventions relate to the initial uptake of exercise. To overcome this, short-term 'introductory periods' can be used, providing high levels of support to small groups of new service users, perhaps from dedicated exercise staff. However, initial accompaniment to exercise should be geared towards gradually stepped-down support, leading people towards autonomy within their own exercise routines sustained through encouragement from care teams and peer support.

---

## KEY MESSAGE 7.7

Delivering exercise through community leisure services has an array of practical and social benefits:

- These services offer discounted rates to service users, and free access to their carers, for a broad range of facilities and activities, accommodating all preferences.
- Community leisure centres are generally centrally located and well served by public transport, making them very accessible.
- Community interventions reduce stigma, promote positive social reintegration, and are continuously available to service users even after/outside of mental health care.

---

It should also be considered that the exercise preferences of people with early psychosis may differ from older people with longer-term mental health problems, who tend to prefer low-intensity activities such as walking (Browne et al., 2015). This may be due to people with early psychosis being fitter, younger and less likely to be held back by obesity and other physical health problems. Nonetheless, the In-Shape study (Bartels et al., 2013) showed that, given appropriate levels of intensity, even people with enduring mental health problems can be engaged with individualised gym-based training. However, community leisure services often offer an array of other exercise options (including walking groups, fitness classes or swimming) that might be better suited for some service users.

Regardless of how the intervention is delivered, various 'behavioural change techniques' can also be applied to bolster motivation. The specific motivational techniques applied within iBEEP were based on established effective techniques for physical activity behaviour change (Greaves et al., 2011; Michie et al., 2011b). These included 'action planning', 'goal-setting' and 'self-monitoring', and were incorporated into the paper-based resources that we provided to participants. First, our 'Exercise Log Book' (available online) was completed by research assistants and service users together, to set action plans and goals at the beginning of the programme, and subsequently track their own progress towards these over time. It is important to remember that attendance-based goals (e.g. aiming to attend twice per week) may be more achievable and motivating than other outcome goals such as weight loss, which are strongly influenced by other factors. Second, the 'Any-Exercise Calendar' (available online) was provided to participants after they finished the 10-week intervention in order to aid them in their efforts to continue exercising at least twice per week, through self-monitoring attendance in a simple, yet structured, format.

## CONCLUSION

Despite the many benefits of exercise, people with mental health problems experience various barriers towards physical activity. In order to overcome these, exercise interventions should be tailored to personal incentives, preferences and circumstances. Furthermore, exercise should be implemented as early as possible, when people are young, fitter and more readily engaged with moderate-to-vigorous activities. Such interventions may also be more effective at this stage, to prevent weight gain, metabolic dysfunction and enduring functional disability from arising (see Chapter 6).

The iBEEP intervention showed that an individualised approach enables people with early psychosis to achieve sufficient amounts of weekly exercise. Furthermore, we observed significant improvements in physical health, symptoms and cognitive functioning after just 10 weeks. Along with several similar trials, results suggest that tailored gym-training programmes are engaging and effective for people with mental health problems. Making use of community leisure resources can increase the feasibility of the implementation and maintenance of exercise overtime. Such interventions could significantly reduce cardiometabolic risk and improve functional recovery.

## USEFUL RESOURCES

*Note*: No copyright is attached. All resources can be used free of charge.

Any-Exercise Calendar Available at: file:///C:/Users/Tim/AppData/Local/Temp/4)%20Any-Exercise%20Calendar.pdf (accessed 5 August 2016).

A simplified exercise recording system to be completed by the service user, promoting at least twice-weekly exercise.

Exercise Formulation Questionnaire website. Available at: file:///C:/Users/Tim/AppData/Local/Temp/1)%20iBeep%20Exercise%20Formulation.pdf (accessed 5 August 2016).

A standardised questionnaire used for developing service users' personalised exercise programmes.

Exercise Log Book. Available at: file:///C:/Users/Tim/AppData/Local/Temp/3)%20Training%20Log%20Book.pdf (accessed 5 August 2016).

A 10-week exercise logbook to record types, frequency and duration of exercise, along with tracking progress towards short- and long-term goals.

Investigating the Benefits of Exercise in Early Psychosis (iBEEP) Exercise Guide website. Available at: www.researchgate.net/publication/299468462_2_IBEEP_Gym-training_guide (accessed 5 August 2016).

Training guides for two alternative gym sessions with cardiovascular and resistance training exercises.

## ANSWERS TO MULTIPLE CHOICE QUESTIONS

1(d), 2(d), 3(c), 4(c), 5(c), 6(a), 7(c), 8(c), 9(a), 10(d)

# EIGHT

## SMOKING CESSATION

### TIM BRADSHAW

## CHAPTER LEARNING OUTCOMES

After reading this chapter, you will be able to:

- Compare the prevalence of smoking in people with mental health problems with other members of the general population.
- Review the harmful effects of smoking and the benefits of quitting.
- Consider the main reasons why so many people with mental health problems smoke.
- Examine barriers to giving up smoking for people with mental health problems.
- Describe an effective evidence-based smoking cessation intervention for people with mental health problems.

## MULTIPLE CHOICE QUESTIONS

We have included 10 multiple choice questions at the beginning of this chapter for readers wishing to test their knowledge of its contents. We have included the answers at the end of the chapter, but advise you not to check these until you have answered them before and after reading the chapter so that you can determine how much your knowledge has increased.

1. Approximately what percentage of the adult population of England smoke?

   a) 19%
   b) 33%
   c) 15%
   d) 45%

2. Approximately what percentage of adults with any form of mental health problem living in England smoke?

   a) 20%
   b) 33%
   c) 15%
   d) 45%

*(Continued)*

*(Continued)*

3. One year after stopping smoking, what benefits can a person expect?

   a) Improvements in respiratory, cardiovascular and reproductive health.
   b) Improvements in mental health, including lower levels of anxiety and depression.
   c) Better social networks and more friends.
   d) All of the above.

4. Between 2000 and 2050, how many deaths is it estimated will be attributed globally to smoking?

   a) 10.5 million.
   b) 450 million.
   c) 90 million.
   d) 250 million.

5. What percentage of premature deaths did Brown et al. (2010) attribute to smoking-related diseases in a group of 350 people with schizophrenia?

   a) 70%
   b) 25%
   c) 50%
   d) 90%

6. What reasons have been suggested for why people with mental health problems are more likely to smoke than others in the general population?

   a) Boredom.
   b) Self-medication.
   c) Culture of mental health services.
   d) All of the above.

7. Which of the following statements about the relationship between antipsychotic medication and smoking is true:

   a) There is no relationship between the dosage of medication required and smoking.
   b) Service users who smoke require lower doses of medication as it helps to relieve stress.
   c) Service users who smoke are generally less compliant with medication.
   d) Service users who smoke require higher doses of medication.

8. If a person wants to stop smoking, how much will the correct combination of pharmacological and behavioural support increase their chances of success?

   a) They will be twice as likely to quit.
   b) They will be five times more likely to quit.
   c) They will be four times more likely to quit.
   d) They will be ten times more likely to quit.

9. What is the most effective way to use Nicotine Replacement Therapy (NRT)?

   a) As a quick mist spray.
   b) By using a combination of gum and spray.
   c) As a nasal spray.
   d) By using a combination of slow release patches and a quicker release product such as gum.

10. Approximately what percentage of people with serious mental illness express a desire to give up smoking when asked?

   a) 50%
   b) 10%
   c) 25%
   d) 70%

# INTRODUCTION

Approximately 19% of the adult population of England smoke (Niblett, 2015), compared to 33% of those with mental health problems (McManus et al., 2010). It is widely acknowledged that smoking cigarettes is the biggest cause of preventable death in Western society (Muller et al., 2016) and that it contributes significantly to premature mortality in people with mental health problems (Brown et al., 2010). Stopping smoking is the single most significant change that a person can make to their behaviour to improve their health, wellbeing and life expectancy.

Stopping smoking at any age has numerous benefits for physical and mental health as well as promoting enhanced overall wellbeing and better financial status (Shahab, 2013). Yet, mental health professionals have been shown to have negative attitudes towards the ability of people with mental health problems to give up smoking (Dwyer et al., 2009) and mainstream smoking cessation services do not cater well for their needs (McNally and Ratschen, 2010).

A recent report by Action on Smoking and Health (ASH, 2016) has set ambitious targets for the prevalence of smoking in people with mental health problems to decrease to 5% by 2035. ASH (2016) have outlined '12 Ambitions' in order to help them achieve this target, which include: Ambition 3 – staff working in all mental health settings see reducing smoking amongst service users as part of their core role; and Ambition 8 – all inpatient and community mental health sites are smoke-free by 2018. Clearly, helping service users to stop smoking is becoming an increasingly important part of the role of all mental health professionals.

In this chapter, we examine evidence regarding the high prevalence of smoking in people with mental health problems, the reasons why so many of them smoke and the detrimental effects of smoking on their physical and mental health. The chapter will conclude by discussing effective evidence-based approaches for helping people with mental health problems to stop smoking including a bespoke smoking cessation intervention developed specifically for people with serious mental illness that has been evaluated in a recent clinical trial (Gilbody et al., 2015).

# PREVALENCE OF SMOKING IN PEOPLE WITH MENTAL HEALTH PROBLEMS

Figure 8.1 shows that people who experience any type of mental health problem are much more likely to smoke than other members of the general population, with the highest rates being amongst individuals with complex and long-term mental health needs such as substance abuse and psychosis.

Individuals with mental health problems are more likely than others to smoke even before their mental health problems begin (Carney, 2016). Indeed, a recent high-quality systematic review suggested that there might even be a link between daily tobacco use and increased risk of psychosis (Gurillo et al., 2015). People with mental health problems start smoking at a younger age than others (Myles et al., 2012), they smoke more cigarettes per day, they inhale more deeply and they have higher levels of nicotine dependency (Royal College of Physicians, 2013), making it even harder for them to stop smoking than others in the general population. A study by McManus et al. (2010) concluded that 42% of all cigarettes consumed in England are smoked by people with a diagnosable mental disorder.

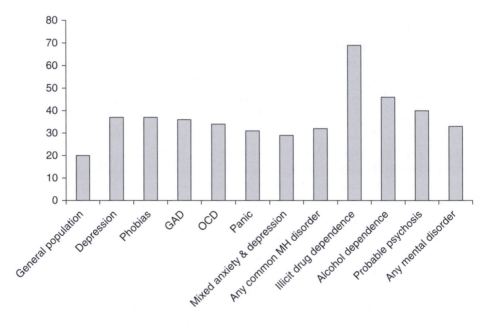

**Figure 8.1    Smoking rate by mental disorder**

*Source*: McManus et al. (2010), reproduced with kind permission of the National Centre for Smoking Cessation and Training (NCSCT)

---

### ⚙ REFLECTION POINT 8.1

Why do you think people with mental health problems are more likely to smoke than other members of the general population?

   Write down your answers and then consider what the evidence shows as you read through this chapter.

# HARMFUL EFFECTS OF SMOKING AND BENEFITS OF GIVING UP

The many harmful effects of smoking on physical health have been summarised by Smokefree NHS on their website (www.nhs.uk/smokefree/why-quit/smoking-health-problems). It can be seen that smoking potentially has detrimental effects on almost all body systems. However, what is less well known is that smoking is not just bad for a person's physical health but may also have a negative impact on their mental health (Shahab, 2013). Many smokers believe that smoking reduces their stress levels and helps them to relax (Shahab and West, 2012). In fact, Jamal et al. (2012) found that symptoms of depression, anxiety and agoraphobia were all more severe in nicotine addicted smokers compared to those who had never smoked, whilst a report by Shahab (2013) showed higher levels of happiness and lower levels of depression and anxiety in people one year after they stopped smoking.

The good news is that many of the harmful effects of smoking on mental and physical health can be avoided and reversed if a person stops smoking. The National Centre for Smoking Cessation and Training (NCSCT) publication *Quick Wins: The Short-Term Benefits of Stopping Smoking* (Shahab, 2013), provides a summary of the numerous benefits that can be gained within one year of stopping smoking, and is summarised in Table 8.1.

Shahab concludes that:

> up to 90% of excess mortality caused by smoking can be prevented if smokers stopped before they reached middle age but even people who have smoked most of their lives can still expect substantial health benefits when they stop smoking. (Ibid.: 5)

**Table 8.1   Improvements in health and wellbeing within one year of stopping smoking**

| | |
|---|---|
| Physical health gains | Improvements in respiratory, vascular, reproductive and gastrointestinal health |
| Mental health gains | Higher levels of happiness and lower levels of depression and anxiety |
| Aesthetic improvements | Improvements in oral health such as bad breath, stained teeth and periodontal disease |
| | Improved appearance of skin and nails |
| Psychosocial benefits | Higher self-confidence (or self-efficacy) and greater internal locus of control Better social networks and friendships |
| Improvements in other health behaviours | Healthy lifestyle changes such as increases in exercise, healthy dieting, reduction in alcohol consumption and taking part in health-screening programmes |
| Financial gains | Based on a smoking habit of 20 cigarettes per day at a cost of £8.50 a packet, a person would save on average £3,102.50 per year |

*Source*: Shahab (2013), reproduced with kind permission of the National Centre for Smoking Cessation and Training (NCSCT)

# CONTRIBUTION OF SMOKING TO EXCESS MORTALITY

On average, smokers die 10 years earlier than non-smokers, with the principle causes of death being vascular, neoplastic and respiratory diseases (Doll et al., 2004). Prabhat (2009) estimates that, globally, between 2000 and 2050, approximately 450 million people will be killed by smoking, with at least half dying between the ages of 30 and 69.

Unsurprisingly, given the high prevalence of smoking in people with mental health problems, it has been shown to be a major contributory factor to excess mortality in this population (Brown et al., 2010). One large epidemiological study in the USA concluded that tobacco-related conditions accounted for 53% of all deaths in hospital patients with schizophrenia, 48% in bipolar disorder and 50% in people with depression (Callaghan et al., 2014). In contrast, a 25-year follow-up study of 350 people with serious mental illness conducted in Southern England found that of the 289 people who had died, 70% of the deaths were attributable to smoking-related diseases (Brown et al., 2010).

# WHY DO PEOPLE WITH MENTAL HEALTH PROBLEMS SMOKE?

Reasons for the high prevalence of smoking in people with mental health problems include using cigarettes as self-medication (McCloughen., 2003), the culture of mental health services (Jochelson and Majrowski, 2006) and boredom (Peckham et al., 2015).

## *SELF-MEDICATION*

We have already mentioned that many people in the general population who smoke believe that smoking cigarettes relieves tension and helps them to relax. These beliefs are also held by over 90% of people with serious mental health problems who smoke (ibid.). Therefore, one of the reasons why people with mental health problems smoke seems likely to be as a form of self-medication to help them to relax and manage their stress levels. This is, of course, a misconception as we have already stated that smoking is actually bad for people's mental health and what smokers are actually doing when they have a cigarette is feeding their nicotine addiction, thereby avoiding the unpleasant effects of withdrawal.

## *CULTURE OF MENTAL HEALTH SERVICES*

Historically, both service users and staff in mental health services have been more likely to smoke than others in the general population (Johnson et al., 2009), and staff would often smoke with service users (Lawn, 2004). Cigarettes were used by mental health staff to pacify distressed service users or given out as rewards for them carrying out activities that were requested by staff (such as taking exercise; Thyer and Irvine, 1984). Attitudinal studies have shown that nurses defend the rights of their service users to smoke (Dwyer et al., 2009) and a recent survey of more than 100 mental health nursing staff in New Zealand showed that about half of them still believed that smoking was helpful in the creation of therapeutic relationships (Connolly et al., 2013). Thus, it appears that the denormalisation of smoking that has occurred over the past 20 years in the general population has not been reflected within the culture of mental health services.

## SMOKING AS SOMETHING TO DO

People with serious mental illness have rates of unemployment that are as high as 90% (Marwaha et al., 2007), and they often lack meaningful daytime activity. A recent study by Peckham et al. (2015) compared the reasons why people with serious mental illness smoked with those of other smokers in the general population. The researchers found that 86% of people with serious mental illness reported smoking *gave them something to do* as a reason for smoking, compared to only 19.6% reporting this as a reason in general population smokers (Fidler and West, 2009), suggesting that boredom is, indeed, a confounding influence on smoking in this client group.

---

### ⚙ REFLECTION POINT 8.2

Do you think that the service users you work with would be interested in stopping smoking if help was offered? If they did want to quit, would you feel optimistic about their chances of success and would you consider yourself adequately skilled to help them?

---

# DO PEOPLE WITH MENTAL HEALTH PROBLEMS WANT TO STOP SMOKING AND CAN THEY BE HELPED TO DO SO?

Research suggests that approximately 50% of people with mental health problems who smoke would like to stop if help was available (Jochelson and Majrowski, 2006). A systematic review by Banham and Gilbody (2010) showed that the same approaches to smoking cessation that are effective with other members of the population also work well for people with mental health problems and that, in individuals who are stable, the interventions do not adversely affect their mental health. However, a survey of conventional NHS stop smoking services by McNally and Ratschen (2010) concluded that they did not operate appropriate procedures for supporting the needs of people with mental health problems. A recent pilot study named Smoking Cessation in Mental Ill health Trial (SCIMITAR) showed the effectiveness of a bespoke smoking cessation intervention designed specifically for people with serious mental illness and delivered by mental health professionals (Gilbody et al., 2015). Qualitative evaluation of service users and smoking cessation practitioners' views of the SCIMITAR intervention showed that they valued the bespoke approach and the fact that it was delivered by someone with knowledge of mental health issues (Knowles et al., 2016).

---

⚙ **REFLECTION POINT 8.3**

Whilst working in mental health services, have you noticed any difference in the attitudes of staff and patients towards smoking compared to other people whom you know away from work?

How often have you observed mental health professionals asking patients about their smoking and offering to help them to stop smoking?

---

## BARRIERS TO SMOKING CESSATION IN MENTAL HEALTH SETTINGS

Mental health practitioners may be the most appropriate professionals to deliver smoking cessation interventions to people with mental health problems (ibid.). However, barriers to them fulfilling this role have been shown to exist. We commented earlier on smoking being part of the culture of mental health services. Studies have consistently shown that mental health staff are more likely to be smokers themselves than others in the general population (Johnson et al., 2009; Ratschen et al., 2009). Staff who do smoke express opinions that it is a service user's right to smoke (Dwyer et al., 2009), that staff should be allowed to smoke with them (Dickens and Stubbs, 2004), and that smoking assists the formation of therapeutic relationships (Dwyer et al., 2009; Connolly et al., 2013). Ratschen et al. (2009) also found that only 42% of mental health staff thought helping service users to stop smoking was their responsibility, 50% said that they could not make time for this activity and that staff lacked knowledge about tobacco dependency and its treatment. Perhaps most worryingly, 41% of psychiatrists were unaware that smoking can decrease blood levels of antipsychotic medication and 36% were unaware that stopping smoking could reduce the dosage needed (Ratschen et al., 2009). Without appropriate management of some medications in smoking cessation, toxicity can develop (Campion et al., 2014).

Such negative attitudes and lack of knowledge towards smoking cessation are clearly a barrier to helping service users to give up smoking and we would argue that they are completely unacceptable, given the harmful effects of smoking on health. Indeed, NICE (2013c: p. 48) has published guidelines on 'smoking cessation in secondary care: acute, maternity and mental health services', recommending, amongst other things: (1) that staff-supervised and staff-facilitated smoking breaks are prohibited; (2) that staff, contractor and volunteer contracts do not allow smoking during work hours or when recognisable as an employee (for example, when in uniform, or wearing identification, or handling hospital business); and (3) to ensure that smoking cessation training is completed and updated annually by all mental health staff as part of NHS mandatory training (for example, training provided by the NCSCT). It seems clear from the NICE (ibid.) guidelines that helping service users to stop smoking is the responsibility of all mental health care staff working in secondary care settings and that nurses and other mental health staff should develop the knowledge and skills necessary to perform this role effectively. In the next section of this chapter, we will explore how effective smoking cessation therapy can be delivered to this client group.

# TRAINING IN SMOKING CESSATION THERAPY

The NCSCT provides a range of evidence-based online training programmes on its website that can be accessed and completed free of charge by health care professionals. The training developed by the NCSCT is underpinned by evidence from research (Michie et al., 2011a) that identifies the competencies (skills and knowledge) that are required by smoking cessation practitioners and behaviour change techniques that the evidence suggests are most effective in helping smokers to quit.

Most of the training is designed with smokers in the general population in mind, however there are also specialist training programmes for people from high-risk groups such as pregnant woman and people with mental health problems.

## *VERY BRIEF ADVICE*

The most basic level of training offered by the NCSCT is called *very brief advice*. This can be used opportunistically in any health care interaction and takes less than

30 seconds to deliver. Research shows that offering very brief advice to all smokers is much more effective in prompting a quit attempt than advising smokers to quit and offering assistance only to those who express an interest in quitting (Aveyard et al., 2012). Very brief advice involves the use of the 3 As: (1) **Ask** about current smoking status; (2) **Advise** the smoker that the most effective way to stop smoking is with a combination of behavioural and pharmacological support; and (3) **Act** if the smoker is interested in making a quit attempt by referring them or signposting them to an evidence-based smoking cessation service.

---

⚙ **REFLECTION POINT 8.4**

The online NCSCT 'very brief advice' training can be completed in less than 30 minutes. If you haven't previously completed the training, we recommend that you go online at: http://elearning.ncsct.co.uk/vba-launch and complete it today.

---

## THE NATIONAL CENTRE FOR SMOKING CESSATION AND TRAINING (NCSCT) TRAINING AND ASSESSMENT PROGRAMME

The NCSCT Stage 1 training programme takes 6–8 hours to complete online in one sitting and contains information about: (1) smoking in the population; (2) smoking and health; (3) why stopping smoking can be difficult; (4) smoking cessation treatments; and (5) the wider context. The training programme contains evidence-based information but also video clips explaining and demonstrating important components of behavioural support. There are self-test questions in most sections for practitioners to be able to assess their own knowledge as they progress. On completion, an 'assessment' consisting of 24 multiple choice questions can be taken. If the pass mark of 70% is achieved, an NCSCT Level 1 certified stop smoking cessation practitioner certificate is awarded. If the practitioner fails to achieve a pass in the assessment, they can sit the test again after a minimum of seven days to allow them to read through the training programme again.

Stage 2 training in behavioural support is also available from the NCSCT and is delivered as a two-day face-to-face training programme (availability and costs on application to the NCSCT). This allows practice to be assessed through role plays, in addition to assessing knowledge. On completion of Stage 2 training, practitioners achieve full NCSCT certification.

## MENTAL HEALTH SPECIALITY MODULE

The NCSCT Mental Health Speciality Module is intended for anyone who works with smokers with mental health issues. The online training module contains information about the relationship between mental health and smoking and advice about how to support people with mental health problems either to make a quit attempt or to 'Cut Down to Quit'. The training includes information about how to safely prescribe pharmacological support and manage the dosage of psychiatric medication; it also discusses how practitioners can manage issues such as service users who want to use e-cigarettes as a substitute to smoking. Completing this module is invaluable for mental health workers who have a role in supporting service users in trying to cut down or quit smoking.

## EFFECTIVE SMOKING CESSATION INTERVENTIONS

Despite numerous advertising campaigns promoting the effectiveness of smoking cessation services, it is perhaps surprising that many people who try to give up smoking do so without professional help by going 'cold turkey'. Yet, research suggests that a quit attempt is twice as likely to succeed if pharmacological support is prescribed (Stead et al., 2012), and four times more likely to succeed if both pharmacological and behavioural support are offered from an appropriately trained practitioner (ibid., 2015). Therefore, any smoker who wants to try and stop smoking should be offered a combination of both treatments.

## NCSCT STANDARD TREATMENT PROGRAMME

The NCSCT standard treatment programme recommends that both pharmacological and behavioural smoking cessation support is delivered over a 5–6 week period. This starts with a pre-quit assessment, where a structured agenda is followed to assist the practitioner to gather information about the person's smoking history and to share information with them that will help enhance their motivation to quit, e.g.: 'Your chances of quitting are much better if you use a combination of behavioural support, from a trained stop smoking practitioner, and an effective stop smoking medication compared with going "cold turkey" (NCSCT, 2014: 8). At the end of the pre-quit session, preparations for quitting are made such as obtaining the correct pharmacological support and knowing how to use it properly, then a quit date is set which is normally 1–2 weeks later. At this and all subsequent meetings, a carbon monoxide (CO) reading is taken and the importance of complete abstinence ('*not one puff*') is emphasised once the quit date is reached.

The next meeting is normally on the quit date. At this meeting, the service user's motivation to quit is reaffirmed and preparations for quitting (e.g. adequate supply of Nicotine Replacement Therapy or NRT) are checked. The practitioner discusses coping with withdrawal symptoms and high-risk situations and the smoker is encouraged to throw away any remaining cigarettes and smoking-related items such as ash trays and to restate their commitment to quit.

Subsequent sessions over the next four weeks focus on checking the service user's progress, giving positive reinforcement where appropriate, making sure they continue to use pharmacological support properly, dealing with cravings and withdrawal effects and managing high risk situations.

## PHARMACOLOGICAL SUPPORT

The most commonly used pharmacological products available to assist smoking cessation are NRT and atypical antidepressant products such as Verenicline (Champix) or Bupropion (Zyban).

Nicotine Replacement Therapy (NRT) helps reduce the craving for nicotine when making a quit attempt by providing pure nicotine without the other harmful chemicals in cigarettes. NRT may be taken in a number of different formats and via several different routes, such as chewing gum, lozenges, mouth spray, etc. NRT has no known adverse effects.

Service users should be asked if they have used NRT before and if they have, which type they used and how helpful they found it. If they have a preference for a particular form of NRT, then this should guide prescribing, however whichever type they choose they should be informed that evidence suggests using two forms of NRT is more effective than one. For example, most people should be advised to use a long acting patch which slowly releases nicotine through the day (and night if a 24-hour patch is used), but that this should also be supplemented by one of the more rapid release products such as gum or nasal spray. Whichever type of NRT is selected it is important to make sure that the service user knows how to use it properly, for example when using gum it is necessary to chew it every 30 minutes then park it between the lip and gum where the nicotine is absorbed. If the service user is not aware of this they are likely to chew and swallow, which will be ineffective in absorbing nicotine and is also likely to lead to heartburn.

Verenicline (Champix) or Bupropion (Zyban) are taken orally and reduce the desire to smoke. Both medications should be started at least 7 days (and up to 14 days) before the quit date. Common side effects include nausea, headaches and insomnia and Bupropion is contraindicated in people with epilepsy and bipolar disorder due to the risk of seizures (Campion et al., 2014). There have also been reports of neuropsychiatric side effects for both Bupropion and Champix and it is advised that care should be taken when prescribing them for people with a history of mental health problems (ibid.).

If the service user says that they don't want to use medication, then they should be informed that their chances of quitting are doubled if it is used and they should be encouraged to reconsider this decision. Reasons for not wanting to use smoking cessation medications should be explored and any incorrect beliefs challenged. Common misconceptions about NRT include that it is addictive and harmful.

In fact, there are no known serious side effects from NRT and it is important that this is explained to the service user. They should also be advised to keep using it for at least 8 weeks after the quit attempt as stopping it sooner than this will make a lapse more likely.

---

⚙️ **REFLECTION POINT 8.5**

Think about the service users whom you work with: is there anything about them or their lifestyles that might make it harder for them to stop smoking than other smokers in the general population? What additional support do you think they might need to help them to quit?

---

# A BESPOKE SMOKING CESSATION INTERVENTION FOR PEOPLE WITH SERIOUS MENTAL ILLNESS

As mentioned earlier, people with serious mental illness tend to be more highly addicted to nicotine compared to other smokers. Also, because of the smoking culture of mental health services, they are exposed to more high-risk situations when other people will be smoking cigarettes around them. Added to this, they may have problems with concentration, memory and motivation, all of which may potentially hamper efforts to stop smoking. These complications suggest that, in addition to the NCSCT standard treatment programme for smoking cessation recommended for smokers in the general population, people with mental health problems may need a more intensive package of support. In the final section of this chapter, we will describe a bespoke smoking cessation intervention that we developed for people with serious mental illness and then evaluated in a pilot randomised controlled trial called Smoking Cessation in Mental Ill health Trial (SCIMITAR). The results of the SCIMITAR trial showed that over a third of the participants who received the bespoke intervention had stopped smoking at 12 months' follow-up (Gilbody et al., 2015).

---

👥 **CASE STUDY 8.1**

Harriet is a 72-year-old woman who has had a diagnosis of bipolar disorder since she was 30. She has been smoking for over 40 years, and currently smokes 20 cigarettes a day but has noticed that she is getting increasingly short of breath when walking and has decided she would

*(Continued)*

*(Continued)*

like to stop. Harriet is motivated to quit smoking and is happy to agree a quit date but she is worried about whether she will be able give up because she lives in sheltered accommodation with six other residents, all of whom smoke, including her best friend who visits her several times a day.

   Think about the issues facing Harriet in trying to stop smoking. How would you be able to help her to increase her chances of a successful quit attempt?

As stated above, the SCIMITAR intervention was based on the NCSCT standard treatment programme but has been modified in a number of ways:

1. The intervention was delivered by practitioners who were experienced in working with people with serious mental health problems but who were also trained as Level 2 NCSCT accredited smoking cessation therapists.
2. The intervention was more intensive than the one described in the NCSCT standard treatment programme; home visits were offered when requested and up to 10 sessions of support were provided.
3. The use of NRT was encouraged, rather than Verenicline or Bupropion, and participants were encouraged to use more than one type of NRT and informed that they could continue to use it for as long as they wanted to.
4. Special attention was paid to medication management (see below). If participants were prescribed certain antipsychotic medication, the smoking cessation practitioners worked closely with prescribers to titrate doses to appropriate levels (Campion et al., 2014). Procedures followed will be described in more detail below. The fact that it was likely that medication doses could be reduced was perceived as an additional incentive to give up smoking by many service users and was used by the smoking cessation practitioners to reinforce their motivation to quit.
5. Finally, for participants who thought that setting an immediate quit date was anxiety-provoking, an alternative approach known as 'Cut Down to Quit' was offered. With Cut Down to Quit, the service user is encouraged to start NRT (pre-load) before reducing the number of cigarettes they smoke each day, then a programme for systematic reduction is worked out with a view to setting a quit date in the near future.

## MEDICATION MANAGEMENT AND SMOKING CESSATION

The production of an enzyme in the liver, CYP 1A2, is stimulated by the polycyclic aromatic hydrocarbons found in tobacco smoke (Rawlinson and Bradshaw, 2014). This increases the metabolism of some medications, including antidepressants (tricyclics and mirtazapine), antipsychotics (clozapine, olanzapine and haloperidol) and benzodiazepines, meaning that smokers require higher doses of medication to achieve similar therapeutic effects. This has important implications for smoking cessation interventions in people taking these medications because, when they stop smoking, plasma levels may rise to potentially toxic levels.

To assist prescribers in the safe management of these drugs in people wanting to quit smoking, the Royal College of Psychiatrists (Campion et al., 2014) has produced a very helpful set of guidelines. It recommends that blood levels of service users prescribed clozapine or olanzapine should be checked prior to the quit date, that doses should be reduced by 25% during the first week of cessation and that further blood tests should be taken on a weekly basis until levels stabilise. Advice about managing other types of medication is also provided.

## CONCLUSION

The prevalence of smoking in people with mental health problems is much higher than in the general population and up to half of all premature deaths in this client group can be attributed to the effects of smoking related diseases. Smoking has for a long time been part of the culture of mental health services and systematic barriers exist for service users who wish to stop smoking. Despite this, evidence suggests that approximately half of the people with mental health problems who smoke would like to try and quit if help was available. In this chapter, we argued that helping people with mental health problems to stop smoking is an important part of the role of nurses and other mental health professionals. We described training that is available to deliver smoking cessation interventions and we outlined how the NCSCT standard treatment programme may be delivered more flexibly to help meet the specific needs of smokers with mental health problems.

## USEFUL RESOURCES

National Centre for Smoking Cessation and Training (NCSCT), Mental Health and Smoking Cessation Specialty Module. Available at: http://elearning.ncsct.co.uk/mental_health_specialty_module-registration (accessed 4 August 2016).

This module focuses on the needs of people who have been diagnosed with a mental health problem who wish to stop smoking. The module introduces practitioners to issues that are specific to the needs of this client group and, in our opinion, together with the NCSCT training and assessment programme, it should be completed by any practitioner who intends to help people with mental health problems to stop smoking.

NCSCT, Training and Assessment Programme. Available at: www.ncsct.co.uk/publication_training-and-assessment-programme.php (accessed 4 August 2016).

This online training programme allows stop smoking practitioners to demonstrate that they have core knowledge and skills to deliver effective behavioural support to people trying to stop smoking. It should be completed by anyone who is in a role where they help smokers to stop smoking.

NCSCT, *Very Brief Advice on Smoking*. Available at: http://elearning.ncsct.co.uk/vba-stage_1 (accessed 4 August 2016).

This evidence-based online course takes less than half an hour to complete and can be used to significantly increase the chances of a smoker agreeing to make a quit attempt. We strongly recommend that all readers of this book complete it.

Royal College of General Practitioners (RCGP) (2014) *Primary Care Guidance on Smoking and Mental Disorders* (2014 update). Available at: www.rcgp.org.uk/clinical-and-research/toolkits/~/media/E7087878A24547E795903F432738AD35.ashx (accessed 4 August 2016).

This information sheet, endorsed by several royal colleges and public health bodies, was developed to assist professionals who are supporting people with mental health problems to stop smoking. As well as information about smoking and mental health, specific advice is provided about how to manage the dosage of certain psycho-tropic medications during smoking cessation.

## ANSWERS TO MULTIPLE CHOICE QUESTIONS

1(a), 2(b), 3(d), 4(b), 5(a), 6(d), 7(d), 8(c), 9(d), 10(a)

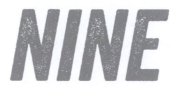

# NINE

## WEIGHT MANAGEMENT

### JACKIE CLEATOR AND TIM BRADSHAW

### CHAPTER LEARNING OUTCOMES

After reading this chapter, you will be able to:

- Describe the prevalence of overweight or obesity in people with mental health problems compared to others in the general population.
- Explore the reasons for weight problems, with particular focus on the obesogenic effects of antipsychotic medication.
- Understand the evidence base for effective weight management interventions.
- Describe an example of an effective intervention that has recently been evaluated in a pilot randomised controlled trial.

### MULTIPLE CHOICE QUESTIONS

We have included 10 multiple choice questions at the beginning of this chapter for readers wishing to test their knowledge of its contents. We have included the answers at the end of the chapter, but advise you not to check these until you have answered them before and after reading the chapter so that you can determine how much your knowledge has increased.

1. Body mass index (BMI) is measured by:

   a) Calculating the degree of weight change over time.
   b) Dividing a person's weight in kilos by their height in metres squared ($kg/m^2$).
   c) Dividing a person's height in metres by their weight in kilos squared ($m/kg^2$).
   d) Assessing the impact of a person's age and gender on their weight.

2. Waist circumference is a useful measure of adiposity as it is:

   a) The most widely accepted measure to assess obesity-related ill health.
   b) An indicator of fat levels around the abdominal organs.
   c) The only way to measure obesity-related ill health in the Caucasian population.
   d) Easily estimated, just by looking at the client.

*(Continued)*

*(Continued)*

3. Obesity in people with mental illness is most likely related to:

   a) Lifestyle factors.
   b) Hereditability.
   c) Characteristics of their illness and treatment side effects.
   d) A complex interaction of all of these factors.

4. Ghrelin is a hormone produced by the lining of the stomach. Its role is to:

   a) Stimulate appetite and encourage a person to eat.
   b) Promote satiety by indicating when the stomach is full.
   c) Accelerate the digestion of fatty food.
   d) Provide resistance to harmful bacteria.

5. A recommended level of weight loss which will achieve clinical benefits is:

   a) 1–4%
   b) 2–4%
   c) 5%
   d) 4%

6. Weight gain in young people treated with antipsychotic medication:

   a) Is usually rapid in onset over the first year of treatment and then sustained over time.
   b) Tends to develop gradually, with the highest levels seen after several years of treatment.
   c) Is very rare and not considered a major clinical issue.
   d) Is only a problem if individuals do not take their medication as directed.

7. NICE guidance (2014a: CG178) recommends that:

   a) People with psychosis or schizophrenia, especially those taking antipsychotics, should be offered a combined healthy eating and physical activity programme by their mental health provider.
   b) People who have gained more than 10% of their body weight whilst taking antipsychotics should be prioritised for weight loss surgery.
   c) People with psychosis or schizophrenia, especially those taking antipsychotics, should be encouraged to join a gym.
   d) Antipsychotic medication should be automatically discontinued in individuals who have gained more than 10% of their body weight whilst taking the medication.

8. According to Thomas et al. (2014), the following factors help people maintain weight loss in the long term:

   a) Eating a low carbohydrate diet, undergoing at least one hour of moderate intensity exercise a day, weighing themself regularly.
   b) Eating a low calorie, low fat diet with little variation, eating breakfast every day, weighing themself regularly.
   c) Walking to work, not eating breakfast, avoiding social occasions.
   d) Avoiding social occasions, undergoing at least one hour of moderate-intensity exercise a day, eating breakfast every day.

9. Systematic reviews of the evidence (Bonfioli et al., 2012; Bruins et al., 2014) have shown that non-pharmacological weight-loss interventions for people with psychotic disorders can:

   a) Improve depressive symptoms as well as cardiovascular risk factors.
   b) Improve quality of life but have limited clinical benefits.

c) Improve cardiovascular risk factors but have no impact on mental health problems.

d) Improve attendance at appointments with a dietitian.

10. Key components of an effective weight loss intervention for young people with first-episode psychosis include:

a) Lifestyle advice and support, group objectives and a range of group sporting and leisure activities.

b) Free access to sports facilities, group objectives and access to support groups.

c) Lifestyle advice and support, personal goal-setting and a range of group sporting and leisure activities.

d) Online peer support, social activities and vouchers for low-fat meals.

# INTRODUCTION

There are currently about 2 billion adults worldwide who are either overweight or obese, with this figure set to rise to 2.7 billion by 2025 (WHO, 2016b), a figure that has been described as being of epidemic proportions (Goodwin and Stambolic, 2015). In 2014, a staggering 61.7% of adults in the UK and Ireland were identified as either overweight or obese (Health Survey for England, 2016).

Caught up in this public health catastrophe are people with mental health problems. Evidence has consistently shown that they are even more likely to be overweight or obese than other members of the populations in which they live (Mitchell et al., 2013b; Bradshaw and Mairs, 2014). This has prompted authors such as Bailey et al. to describe the situation as being like '*an epidemic within an epidemic*' (2012: 376).

In this chapter, we will examine evidence regarding how the weight of people with mental health problems compares to others and will consider some of the challenges faced by this client group in trying to control their weight. We will review the evidence base for effective weight management interventions, firstly in the general population and secondly by looking at interventions that have been developed specifically for people with mental health problems. Finally, we will describe the components of an effective weight management intervention developed in a recent study for people with first-episode psychosis that might be used by practitioners in routine practice settings.

# HOW CAN WE MEASURE OVERWEIGHT OR OBESITY?

How a person's weight relates to their health can be determined by calculating their body mass index (BMI). The BMI is calculated by dividing a person's weight in kilograms by their height in metres squared ($kg/m^2$). The WHO (2016b) suggests the following thresholds for adults: $<18.5 \ kg/m^2$ = underweight; $18.5–24.9 \ kg/m^2$ = normal weight; $25.0–29.9 \ kg/m^2$ = overweight; and $30 \ kg/m^2$ and above = obese. These reflect the increasing health risk of excess weight as the BMI increases above an optimal range of $21–23 \ kg/m^2$.

## ACTIVITY 9.1    CALCULATING BMI

John has noticed that he has gained weight recently but is unsure if this is a problem. He is 1.82 metres tall and weighs 97.9 kg. You calculate his BMI to be 29.5 kg/m$^2$ (97.9 kg/1.82 m/1.82 m), indicating that he is overweight:

- What advice would you give him?

Although the BMI can be calculated manually, as in the above example, there are a number of web-based calculators such as the one on the UK NHS Choices website (webwww.nhs.uk/Tools/Pages/Healthyweightcalculator.aspx). This website will not only calculate your BMI classification but will also provide you with advice about how much weight you should try to lose if you are overweight and how to lose it.

- Try visiting the website and working out what your own BMI is.

BMI is a simple measure that is very useful for calculating obesity at a population level, but it is not without limitations. It provides a proxy measure of the total amount of body fat (adiposity) but does not account for the relative proportions of fat and lean tissue in a range of body shapes and cannot identify where fat is located or how the body will respond physiologically to fat storage. It is the fat around abdominal organs (viscera) that presents the highest risk to health and this is more accurately measured through waist circumference, which is considered a reliable marker for visceral fat (Pischon et al., 2008).

Therefore, the WHO (2016b) recommends measuring both the BMI and central adiposity together in order to determine an individual's relative risk of obesity-related ill health, and it has identified a set of thresholds based on levels of BMI and two cut-off points for waist circumference (Table 9.1). Whilst measuring waist circumference is not always practical in vulnerable individuals as it is somewhat invasive, it can be particularly useful for some groups such as people of South Asian origin who are more prone to carrying excess fat centrally rather than peripherally and show raised obesity-related risk at lower BMI and waist circumference levels than Caucasian groups (Hsu et al., 2015).

Table 9.1   World Health Organization classification for risk of obesity-related ill health

| Classification | BMI (kg/m²) | Waist circumference (cm) | |
| --- | --- | --- | --- |
| | Men: | 94–102 | >102 |
| | Women: | 80–88 | >88 |
| Underweight | <18.5 | No increased risk | No increased risk |
| Healthy weight | <18.5–24.9 | No increased risk | Increased risk |
| Overweight | 25–29.9 | Increased risk | High risk |
| Obesity | >30 | High risk | Very high risk |

Source: WHO (2016b), reproduced with kind permission of WHO

# WHY IS IT IMPORTANT TO MEASURE OVERWEIGHT AND OBESITY?

Regardless of how it is measured, evidence consistently shows that being over-weight or obese is associated with an increased risk for a range of common physical health problems. The mechanical effects of excess weight include conditions such as osteoarthritis and obstructive sleep apnoea, and endocrine and cardiovascular effects include heart disease, stroke, hypertension and type 2 diabetes (Guh et al., 2009; Garber, 2012; Vincent et al., 2012; Kuna et al., 2013). Several common can-cers, including breast and bowel cancer, are also known to be weight related (Bhaskaran et al., 2014).

The combined impact of obesity and obesity-related conditions on future well-being is very clear. Prospective studies show that maintaining a BMI of 30–35 kg/m$^2$ equates to 2–4 years of life lost, and a BMI of 40–45 kg/m$^2$ equates to 8–10 years of life lost (Whitlock et al., 2009). Therefore, it is important that health professionals are both monitoring those at risk and helping individuals to achieve weight loss. In Chapters 6 and 10, we outlined the importance of routinely mon-itoring the weight of service users with mental health problems and provided guidance for practitioners about the course of action to take if a service user's BMI is >25 kg/m$^2$.

## KEY MESSAGE 9.1

Overweight and obesity are matters of serious concern, with wide-ranging effects on physical health. As health care professionals, we have a responsibility to identify and explain obesity-related health risk to service users:

- BMI is the most widely accepted tool for measuring overweight and obesity.
- Waist circumference may be a more useful indicator of adiposity, particularly in some non-Caucasian populations.

# CAUSES OF OVERWEIGHT AND OBESITY

Medical causes of obesity range from common conditions where weight gain is usually gradual such as the menopause or hypothyroidism (reduced production of thyroxine), to much rarer conditions such as Cushing's syndrome. In this instance, weight gain is caused by high levels of cortisol and is usually very rapid, particularly around the abdomen. Whilst it is important to exclude these conditions in any individual, obesity experienced by those with mental illness is more likely to be related to other factors such as lifestyle, hereditability, characteristics of their illness, treatment side effects or a complex interaction of all of these factors (Holt and Peveler, 2009).

Modern-day living in both developed and developing countries has seen the emergence of an 'obesogenic' environment (Goodwin and Stambolic, 2015). Low-cost calorie-rich food is increasingly available and the adoption of a more sedentary lifestyle by both children and adults means that 'active' living no longer represents normality (Government Office for Science, 2012). Other changes in lifestyle such as reductions in total sleep time and sleep quality are a further contributing factor. At a population level, the average time asleep has reduced in recent years from 10 hours to 7 hours (Gangwisch et al., 2005). Short sleep times of less than 7 hours are known to be associated with obesity, with the degree of obesity worsening as sleep time gets shorter (Wu et al., 2014).

This 'obesogenic' environment provides an unfortunate backdrop for any individual with a genetic susceptibility to obesity. One in six of the population, for example, are now known to have a variation in the fat mass and obesity associated (FTO) gene, making them 70% more likely to become obese. This is due to higher levels of ghrelin, a hormone produced by the lining of the stomach that stimulates appetite and makes the increased availability of food even harder to resist (van Dijk et al., 2015). For individuals who go on to develop obesity-related conditions such as type 2 diabetes, weight loss becomes even more difficult as most treatments, particularly insulin, result in weight gain (King et al., 1998).

---

**ﾚﾚ   CASE STUDY 9.1**

Camila attends her doctor's surgery, wanting a 'quick-fix diet pill' as she has gained 12 kg in weight over the past two years. She has tried 'every diet under the sun' and nothing has worked. She is very upset and frustrated by this and can't understand why this has happened. She doesn't want to end up like her sister, who is very overweight and struggles to walk. After gentle probing to understand Camila's 'typical day', we discover that she recently went through the menopause; she struggles to fall asleep, worrying about her husband's health; but she still has to get up early to look after her daughter's children. Most days, she takes the children out to McDonald's for lunch so her husband can rest.

---

Bailey et al. (2012) stress that individuals with mental illness are no less likely to experience any of these influencing factors, but face additional challenges caused by their particular condition. Depression is very common in obese populations and there is strong evidence to suggest that the link is bi-directional, with both obesity and depression impacting on each other (Luppino et al., 2010). Commonly pre-scribed antidepressant drugs such as citalopram are also known to cause moderate weight gain (Blumenthal et al., 2014).

However, for young people with psychosis, the effects of psychiatric medications on their weight can be excessive. Many young people commencing treatment with antipsychotic medication gain weight rapidly in the first few months after starting to take the medication (Chapter 6). For example, in a group of 498 first-episode people prescribed olanzapine, Kahn et al. (2008) found that the number classified as being overweight rose from 16% at baseline to 54% after one year, with an average weight gain of 13.9 kg. If not properly managed, this kind of rapid weight gain has been linked to other cardiometabolic disturbances and may be a significant factor in the poor long-term health experienced by this client group (Chapter 6).

Worryingly, there is a dearth of evidence regarding how long weight gain resulting from the prescription of antipsychotic medication is expected to continue, with the vast majority of studies only following up people for a maximum of 12 months (Bradshaw and Mairs, 2014). However, in a three-year follow-up, Addington et al. (2006) found that, although weight gain slowed down after one year post-first episode, participants continued to gain over 2% of their body weight in each of the second and third years of treatment. It appears then that for these young people, the side effects of treatment are devastating, with an emerging picture that weight gain is both rapid and sustained over time.

## ⚙ REFLECTION POINT 9.1

Thinking about your current practice:

- What are your priorities when a service user first starts antipsychotic medication?
- How important is it to explain the side effects of medication at this stage?
- What would you say to the service user about potential weight gain?

# WHY DOES ANTIPSYCHOTIC MEDICATION CAUSE WEIGHT GAIN?

Service users who are prescribed atypical antipsychotic medication often complain of having an increased appetite that is not satisfied even after eating. This is likely to be related to the effects of ghrelin, the hormone that stimulates appetite. Research has shown that individuals prescribed antipsychotic medication such as olanzapine show raised fasting serum ghrelin levels (Esen-Danacı et al., 2008), thus over-stimulating their appetite and promoting binge eating (Kluge et al., 2007). Effects are also seen on the insulin cascade causing alterations to glucose uptake and fat distribution, which, in turn, contribute to the increased risks of developing obesity and related conditions such as type 2 diabetes and cardiovascular disease (Teff and Kim, 2011).

As well as increased appetite and metabolic effects, weight gain may be further compounded by the sedative effects of the medication, which makes it more challenging for people to exercise (Chapter 7). Increasing weight gain further compounds this situation, making physical activity more challenging and adversely affecting both self-confidence and self-esteem: thus, a vicious cycle of inactivity and over-eating may develop (Bradshaw and Mairs, 2014).

Being overweight or obese is therefore a significant problem for many people with mental health problems, which, without appropriate intervention, may be a major contributory factor towards longer-term poor physical health. Indeed, NICE recommends that: 'people with psychosis or schizophrenia, especially those taking antipsychotics, should be offered a combined healthy eating and physical activity programme by their mental healthcare provider' (2014a: CG178, Recommendation 7.2.8.1, p. 170).

## KEY MESSAGE 9.2

Weight gain in the general population usually results from a combination of lifestyle factors and genetic susceptibility. For individuals with mental health problems who also experience the added burdens of weight gain due to their condition and the side effects of treatment, the impact of weight gain can be devastating:

- Many young people commencing treatment with antipsychotic medication gain weight rapidly in the first few months of treatment.
- Weight gain is due to changes in appetite and glucose and lipid metabolism.
- As health professionals, we have a responsibility to ensure that service users have access to a healthy eating and weight loss programme.

# EFFECTIVENESS OF WEIGHT MANAGEMENT INTERVENTIONS

## INTERVENTIONS IN THE GENERAL POPULATION

The most enduring public health message about weight loss, which has been around for some time, is that a loss of 5–10% is an achievable and realistic target (Goldstein, 1992). Current evidence even suggests that 5% is sufficient to improve metabolic function and other risk factors for metabolic disease (Magkos et al., 2016). This is generally best achieved with structured weight management interventions. A systematic review by Williams et al. (2015) of 49 high-quality randomised controlled trials of weight loss interventions conducted with members of the general population (BMI range 26–44 kg/m$^2$) showed that interventions are effective in helping both men and women to lose weight. Furthermore, whilst both dietary and exercise interventions have been shown to be effective, the most effective weight loss interventions are those that include a combination of some moderate degree of energy restriction through reduced calorific intake and the inclusion of exercise for increased energy expenditure.

---

### ⚙ REFLECTION POINT 9.2

Christine is 40 years old and weighs 80 kg (BMI 33.3 kg/m²). She is determined to lose weight and wants to return to her ideal weight of 55 kg (BMI 22.9 kg/m²). She last weighed this on her wedding day, 19 years ago, and can remember everyone telling her how fantastic she looked:

- What concerns might you have about Christine's approach?
- How might you be supportive but at the same time help her set a more realistic target?

---

Pharmacological options to support structured interventions are limited at present, with only one medication (Orlistat) currently available in the UK, either on prescription or over the counter in lower strength form (Alia) with reduced effectiveness. Orlistat acts within the gut to inhibit pancreatic lipase and stop the absorption of excess dietary fat. This is then passed out as loose stool. Despite these unpleasant side effects, it is widely used and tolerated well with a meta-analysis of 10,000 individuals taking Orlistat showing a mean weight loss of 2.9 kg at 12 months (Rucker et al., 2007).

Unfortunately, losing weight is generally easier than maintaining weight loss with most people regaining weight over the longer term (Sumithran and Proietto, 2013). Several physiological changes occur after weight loss, where the body works hard to 'defend' against the loss and regain the weight. Levels of the 'satiety hormone' leptin, (which helps regulate the urge to eat), reduce, thus stimulating eating and hedonistic changes alter perceptions of the sight, smell and taste of food to make it more desirable. Evidence from the National Weight Control Registry (Thomas et al., 2014), the largest ongoing investigation of people who have successfully maintained weight loss, suggest considerable ongoing effort is needed, with successful maintainers reporting eating a low calorie, low-fat diet with little variation, taking breakfast every day, weighing themselves regularly, and undergoing at least one hour of purposeful moderate intensity exercise a day.

---

### 👪 CASE STUDY 9.2

Mario's practice nurse advised him to lose weight as his blood pressure had increased to 150/90 mmHg, despite taking anti-hypertensive medication. After six months of being on a diet, Mario proudly reached his weight loss target of 6 kg. He achieved this mainly by avoiding situations that

*(Continued)*

*(Continued)*

tempted him to overeat, such as going to a restaurant with his wife on Saturdays, and he ate lunch at his desk away from his workmates to avoid the canteen food. He went for a swim three times a week but didn't enjoy it, so was relieved to stop once his goal had been achieved. To celebrate his success, he put the bathroom scales back in their box and took his wife out for a treat. His workmates were pleased to see him again at lunchtime, complaining about his previous anti-social behaviour. Two months later, he has noticed that his clothes are getting tight again and he feels hungrier than ever. He is avoiding getting on the scales and has cancelled his last check-up with the nurse. His wife thinks that he should start swimming again but he'd rather put it off until after his holiday.

On a positive note, there is some evidence to suggest that the benefits of weight loss will persist even if the weight is regained. For example, if a person has diabetes and improves their diabetes control during weight loss, this lowers the health risk from diabetes over time, and those at risk of developing diabetes will reduce their risk and slow down the rate of progression to the disease (Diabetes Prevention Program Research Group, 2009).

## WEIGHT LOSS INTERVENTIONS IN PEOPLE WITH MENTAL HEALTH PROBLEMS

### NON-PHARMACOLOGICAL INTERVENTIONS

Further good news is that weight loss interventions specifically focused on people with mental health problems generally show a positive effect. A systematic review by Bruins et al. (2014) considered evidence from 25 randomised controlled trials of lifestyle interventions and found significant short- and long-term effects in relation to both weight loss and weight gain prevention. Interestingly, Bruins et al. (ibid.) also found that weight loss interventions resulted in significant improvements in depressive symptoms as well as cardiometabolic risk factors, including waist circumference, triglycerides, fasting glucose and insulin. This suggests that such interventions for people with mental health problems have the potential to benefit both their physical and mental health. Similar positive findings regarding the effectiveness of lifestyle interventions have been described in reviews by Bonfioli et al. (2012), Caemmerer et al. (2012) and Fernandez-San-Martin et al. (2014).

### PHARMACOLOGICAL INTERVENTIONS

Whilst lifestyle interventions have obvious benefits for both physical and mental health, it should be acknowledged that there will be a proportion of service users who will struggle to engage in such interventions. Failure to engage often results from reduced social support, low expectations and weight-related stigma (Phelan et al., 2015).

Individuals of low socioeconomic status, particularly women living in areas of deprivation, where obese levels are often highest, can struggle to access suitable services (National Obesity Observatory, 2012). For people with a serious mental illness such as psychosis, who may have the additional barrier of reduced levels of activity and motivation, any one of these factors can have a serious impact on engagement.

---

### ⚙ REFLECTION POINT 9.3

You may have had previous experience in working with service users who were reluctant to engage with weight management programmes:

- What were the main barriers identified?
- What did you do to help them overcome these barriers?

---

Thus, pharmacological products may have a role to play to promote weight loss in this client group. Orlistat may be contraindicated in service users with psychosis as non-concordance with a strict low-fat diet might induce unpleasant side effects and failure to absorb antipsychotic medication. However, other medications may be helpful. A systematic review by Praharaj et al. (2011) of 12 studies showed the mean weight loss for the antidiabetic medication Metformin (which helps to improve insulin sensitivity) to be 5.02 kg over 12 weeks compared to a placebo. Another systematic review, this time by Fiedorowicz et al. (2012), compared studies that had investigated the weight loss properties of four different medications and found Metformin to be most effective. These studies suggest that if the feasibility of lifestyle interventions is poor, then Metformin should be considered as an alternative treatment to promote weight loss.

Therefore, the evidence suggests that there is room for optimism that people with mental health problems who are required to take antipsychotic medication can be protected against the unwanted side effect of weight gain if appropriate tailored intervention is offered that acknowledges the particular challenges they face.

---

### KEY MESSAGE 9.3

A weight loss of 5–10% is a realistic and achievable target that has proven clinical benefits. This is best achieved with structured weight management programmes. A key aspect of such programmes is to teach strategies for maintaining weight loss over time:

- Individuals with serious mental illness may struggle to engage in generic weight management programmes.
- The antidiabetic medication Metformin may be an alternative treatment option for this group.

# DEVELOPING AN EFFECTIVE INTERVENTION TO PROMOTE WEIGHT LOSS

As part of the Healthy Living and Prevention of Early Relapse (HELPER) study, Bradshaw et al. (2012) described the development of a bespoke weight management intervention designed specifically for young people with first episode psychosis. In order to develop the intervention, the authors undertook a review of the literature and conducted qualitative interviews with service users, health professionals and carers to establish what type of intervention would be most acceptable to them (Bradshaw et al., 2012).

The result was the development of an intervention to control weight gain designed specifically for this client group. The content of the intervention has been illustrated in Table 9.2. It consisted of eight individual sessions of lifestyle advice and support delivered by a Support Time Recovery worker. Sessions were offered at a venue, according to the preference of each participant, which was often their home, and lasted an average of 40 minutes each. A manual to guide and support service users was developed specifically for the study and is available from the authors on request. Results of a pilot randomised controlled trial (InterACT – Intervention to encourage Activity, improve diet and control weight gain), showed that it had superior effects for weight loss compared to treatment as usual (Lovell et al., 2014). In particular, the difference in weight between service users prescribed olanzapine or clozapine after 12 months was 4.5 kg lower in the intervention group compared to the control group.

**Table 9.2   The HELPER InterACT Intervention schedule**

| Session number | Content |
| --- | --- |
| *Session 1* | Orientation to the session |
| Introduction to the intervention and identification of health beliefs | Orientation to the intervention (including participant's role, STR workers' role, the patient book and the role of family and friends) |
| | Assess lifestyle and elicit health beliefs. Identify and agree individualised goal |
| | Offer choice and options of the scheduled groups |
| | Ending: Feedback on session, final questions, next appointment |
| *Session 2* | Review goals |
| Developing an action plan for change | Develop a feasible and acceptable action plan (identifying barriers and facilitators to implementation) |
| | Collaboratively plan intervention and next steps of the intervention |
| | Ending: Feedback on session, final questions, next appointment |
| *Sessions 3–5* | Review progress on action plan and implementation steps |
| Implementation of the action plan | Collaboratively plan next steps for implementation and implement action plan |
| | Monitoring progress |
| | Ending: Feedback on session, final questions, next appointment |
| *Sessions 6 and 7* | Review progress (measure progress towards goals) |
| Monitoring success | Review action plan |
| | Ending: Feedback on session, final questions, closure of the session, next steps |

| Session number | Content |
|---|---|
| *Session 8* | Review goals |
| Maintaining the gains | Review progress and plan next steps |
| | Plan next steps |
| | Ending: Feedback on intervention |

---

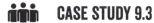 **CASE STUDY 9.3**

Eshal is 21 years old. She is very upset as she has gained 18 kg in eight months after starting olanzapine. Until she became unwell, she had cared a lot about her appearance and hadn't understood what was happening to her at the time of her illness. She knows her mum is worried about her weight, but Eshal feels the situation is hopeless. She prefers not to go out, so can't exercise, she feels hungry all the time and eating passes the time when she is bored at home. Reluctantly, she agreed to see a Support Time Recovery worker about a 'lifestyle intervention'. She was pleasantly surprised when the worker reassured her that she did not need to change everything overnight but could set small targets to aim for each week. As small successes built on each other, Eshal lost 5 kg and gained enough confidence to join a walking group. She has made a friend in the group and they now meet for coffee after the walk has finished.

This case study illustrates the ripple-out effect that such lifestyle interventions may have, not only in terms of promoting weight loss, but also in improving self-confidence and improving social networks. Several service users who participated in the HELPER InterACT study reported similar experiences.

---

### KEY MESSAGE 9.4

Young people with first-episode psychosis experiencing the weight gain effects of treatment will benefit from a bespoke weight management intervention tailored to their specific needs:

- Service users benefit from an identified support worker and individualised goals.
- Home-based interventions are particularly helpful to build confidence in people with low self-esteem.
- A collaborative approach is essential and is maintained throughout the programme.

## CONCLUSION

In this chapter, we considered how the alarming rise of overweight and obesity is becoming a serious global health challenge, as every day we discover yet more harmful effects on physical and psychosocial health. We have argued that health professionals have a particular responsibility to understand this emerging evidence base and to identify and monitor individuals who are most at risk. People with mental health problems are a particularly high-risk group. As well as being exposed to obesogenic lifestyle factors, common to most individuals, they are also at risk of rapid and severe weight gain once they commence treatment with medication. Weight loss for these individuals can seem a daunting prospect, yet there is strong evidence to suggest that a weight loss of 5–10% can be a realistic and achievable target with identified clinical benefits. NICE (2014a: CG178) recommend that this weight loss is best achieved through the supportive environment of a combined healthy eating and physical activity intervention. Yet, for individuals who may experience low self-esteem and social isolation, encouraging them to engage in group-based generic weight management programmes may be counter-intuitive and setting them up for failure. We have made a case, therefore, that the way forward may be to offer bespoke weight management interventions that can be individualised, collaborative at all times and home-based when necessary.

## USEFUL RESOURCES

National Institute for Health and Care Excellence (NICE) (2014) *Obesity: Identification, Assessment and Management of Overweight and Obesity in Children Young People and Adults* (NICE, CG189), report. Available at: www.nice.org.uk/guidance/cg189 (accessed 15 August 2016).

Comprehensive guidance on clinical pathways for individuals with overweight and obesity problems in the UK.

Pearson, D. and Grace, C. (2012) *Weight Management: A Practitioner's Guide*, 1st edn. Ames, IA, Oxford and Chichester: Wiley-Blackwell.

Contains lots of practical advice and uses a stepwise approach to help health care professionals develop skills and gain confidence in weight management.

Public Health England Obesity (n.d.) Available at: www.noo.org.uk/ (accessed 15 August 2016).

Provides a wide range of information on data, evaluation, evidence and research about weight and factors affecting weight gain.

## ANSWERS TO MULTIPLE CHOICE QUESTIONS

1(b), 2(b), 3(d), 4(a), 5(c), 6(a), 7(a), 8(b), 9(a), 10(c)

# TEN

## CONDUCTING HEALTH CHECKS USING THE SERIOUS MENTAL ILLNESS HEALTH IMPROVEMENT PROFILE

### JACQUIE WHITE

## CHAPTER LEARNING OUTCOMES

After reading this chapter, you will be able to:

- Describe the purpose of health screening and provide an example from your own personal health care experience.
- Reflect on your physical health care skills and knowledge as a mental health practitioner and match these to the 28 parameters identified as at most risk in people with serious mental illness.
- Understand how to use the Health Improvement Profile (HIP) and the potential facilitators and enablers to its successful implementation in practice.
- Construct a personal and professional physical health competence action plan.
- Know where to access further information and resources to support implementation of the HIP.

## MULTIPLE CHOICE QUESTIONS

We have included 10 multiple choice questions at the beginning of this chapter for readers wishing to test their knowledge of its contents. We have included the answers at the end of the chapter, but advise you not to check these until you have answered them before and after reading the chapter so that you can determine how much your knowledge has increased.

1. Compared to other members of the general population, people with serious mental illness such as schizophrenia and bipolar disorder:

    a) Are more likely to undergo routine physical health screening.
    b) Are less likely to undergo routine physical health screening.

*(Continued)*

*(Continued)*

    c)  Are just about as likely to undergo routine physical health screening.
    d)  Should have their physical health checked every 5 years.

2. Which of the following best describes the aim of health screening:

    a)  The aim of screening is to detect the prevalence of different health problems in a community.
    b)  The aim of screening is to attempt to identify causal factors for poor health.
    c)  The aim of screening is to facilitate the development of new treatments.
    d)  The aim of screening is to identify health problems early enough to initiate intervention and benefit health outcomes.

3. According to Daumit et al. (2002), compared to other members of the general population, people with serious mental illness:

    a)  Make fewer visits to see their GPs.
    b)  Rarely visit their GP.
    c)  Make more frequent and longer visits to their GP.
    d)  Are often not registered with a GP.

4. How often should the HIP for serious mental illness be completed:

    a)  At lease annually.
    b)  Every month.
    c)  At least every 6 months.
    d)  At each meeting with the service user.

5. How many different parameters of physical health are screened by the HIP?

    a)  28
    b)  12
    c)  21
    d)  18

6. Which of the following findings have surveys of mental health nurses shown:

    a)  They do not think that they should have to provide physical health care to their service users.
    b)  They believe that they are adequately prepared for the role of providing physical health care.
    c)  They think that this is the most important part of their role.
    d)  They lack specific training and confidence to deliver physical health care.

7. What was the finding of White et al.'s (2014) study, which assessed the knowledge of mental health nurses before and after receiving training about the HIP?

    a)  There was no change in their knowledge or attitudes.
    b)  Their attitudes improved but their knowledge was unchanged.
    c)  There was a significant increase in their knowledge.
    d)  There was a significant decrease in their knowledge.

8. Which is the main reason why people with serious mental illness are vulnerable to poor dental health?

    a)  They eat a lot of sweets.
    b)  There is a genetic link between poor dental health and serious mental illness.

   c) They don't clean their teeth often enough.

   d) Antipsychotic medication often causes a dry mouth and therefore reduces the amount of saliva that might protect against decay.

9. The term 'hyperlipidaemia' refers to:

   a) Low levels of circulating lipids in the blood.

   b) Abnormally high levels of circulating lipids in the blood.

   c) Unusually active levels of lipids in the blood.

   d) A rare form of anaemia.

10. If a parameter of the HIP, for example blood pressure, is 'flagged red', which of the following is required:

   a) No further action.

   b) Repeat the assessment in one week's time.

   c) A referral for further investigation/treatment should be made.

   d) The test should be repeated again immediately.

# INTRODUCTION

In this chapter, a risk assessment tool to aid practitioners carrying out physical health checks and interventions is described and the evidence for its implementation in practice to date discussed. The serious mental illness Health Improvement Profile (HIP) was designed to support mental health nurses and other practitioners in their physical health care role.

# HEALTH SCREENING

Health screening in the general population is an integral part of public health policy around the world. The aim of screening is to identify health problems early enough to initiate intervention and benefit health outcomes. Screening can be used to prevent the spread of disease, or exclude people from certain occupations or places. Screening has been defined as:

> the presumptive identification of unrecognised disease or defect by the application of tests, examinations, or other procedures which can be applied rapidly. Screening tests separate out apparently well persons who probably have a disease from those who probably do not. A screening test is not intended to be diagnostic. Persons with positive or suspicious findings must be referred to their physicians for diagnosis and necessary treatment. (Commission on Chronic Illness, 1957: 45)

Some of the earliest health-screening programmes were intended to exclude people with venereal disease, diabetes or psychological disorders from military service in the First World War (Morabia and Zhang, 2004). Life insurance companies in New York implemented mass diabetes screening in 1900. In 1917, tests on drafted and enlisted recruits were implemented to exclude those with 'defective intelligence' from the American army. Between the two World Wars, serological testing for syphilis was implemented for pregnant women (and, in some states of America, for couples intending to marry), certain occupations (for example, army recruits) and on admission to (psychiatric) hospital. Even today, certain communicable diseases or mental illness may exclude people wishing to travel or emigrate to certain countries.

> ## ⚙ REFLECTION POINT 10.1
>
> * What health checks have you personally experienced so far in your life?
> * Think about any health-screening tests you have seen in practice. Think about one where the result was outside the normal range. What action was taken as a result?
> * If your answer to any of the above is 'no' or 'not sure', what can you do to change this?

# HEALTH CHECKS IN PEOPLE WITH SERIOUS MENTAL ILLNESS

Serious mental illness includes people with a diagnosis of schizophrenia, schizo-affective or bipolar disorder. These populations are amongst the least likely in society to have their physical health needs identified and treated and the subsequent and ever-widening mortality gap, compared to people in the general population, has been described as a public health scandal (see Chapters 1 and 2 for more detail about life expectancy in people with serious mental illness).

There is low uptake of public health-screening programmes in people with serious mental illness. A review of 12 studies in the USA, Canada, Australia and Europe concluded that people with serious mental illness were less likely to access cervical, breast, colorectal or prostate screening than other groups (Howard et al., 2010). A systematic review of HIV testing in people with serious mental illness reported a very broad range of lifetime testing rates (11–89%, n=13 studies; Senn and Carey, 2009). Lifetime testing for hepatitis B or C was 41% in 200 service users living in the community in the USA, with no evidence of increased screening or immunisation where high-risk sexual or substance use behaviour was documented (Goldberg et al., 2005). People with co-morbid psychiatric and substance use disorders have been found to have lower rates of immunisation, smoking cessation interventions and cancer screening compared to those with a single serious mental illness diagnosis (Druss et al., 2002). A comparison of screening for metabolic risk parameters in people with serious mental illness compared to those with diabetes from 8123 GP practices in England reported significantly lower rates in those with mental health problems (74.7%, versus 97.3% p<0.001; see Mitchell and Hardy, 2013).

A systematic review of 31 studies concluded that people with mental disorder and/or substance use are less likely to receive recommended treatments (including surgery) for co-morbid diagnoses than controls (that is, in general medicine, cardio-vascular disease, breast cancer and diabetes; Mitchell et al., 2009). In the small number of studies that reported bipolar disorder separately, this disparity was not seen (3 studies). The most recent case linkage study of service users with bipolar disorder registered in primary care in Scotland identified lower than expected rates of treatment (Smith et al., 2013c). People with bipolar disorder and cardiovascular disease and/or hypertension were significantly less likely to be prescribed statins or one or more antihypertensive medicines than controls. These rates do not seem to be associated with problems of access to an appointment and people with serious mental illness are known to make more frequent and longer visits to their GP than general population controls (Daumit et al., 2002).

Disparities in physical health care are known to exist in both hospital and com-munity mental health services in the UK. A baseline audit of records on four randomly selected inpatient wards and one Community Mental Health Team in the largest UK Mental Health NHS Trust identified 100% adult inpatients but only 22% community patients with records of smoking status (Parker et al., 2012). Of the 62 inpatients who reported smoking cigarettes, only 25% had a record of a conversation about risk and only one had been referred to smoking cessation services. For the five cardiometabolic risk factors considered most important in serious mental illness (BMI, blood glucose, lipids, blood pressure and smoking status), the rate for a record of assessment of all five was a disappointing 33% (range 1–77%) in the second National Audit of Schizophrenia (NAS; Royal College of Psychiatrists, 2014). Wide disparity remains between NHS Trusts and inadequate rates of intervention, even where there is a diagnosis of co-morbid physical disease. Selection of community patients with schizophrenia for the NAS is made by the organisation, so may overestimate adherence to the standards as a result of selection bias.

Mental health nurses remain the largest number of health care professionals in secondary care in contact with people with serious mental illness. The equiv-alent group in primary care are (general) practice nurses. Practice nurses arguably have access to more people with a serious mental illness diagnosis than mental health nurses because of the larger population served by GP practices. Both groups of nurses have an opportunity to intervene positively to improve the health of people with serious mental illness through engagement in health screening and intervention.

The Nursing and Midwifery Council require all UK nurses to be competent in a range of 'essential' physical health care skills at the point of registration (Nursing and Midwifery Council, 2010). Despite these standards, surveys of mental health and practice nurses report that they feel poorly equipped for this role in terms of their knowledge, skills and confidence. Surveys of mental health nurses describe motivation to intervene positively in physical health but a lack of specific training and confidence to deliver physical health care (Howard and Gamble, 2011; Robson et al., 2013). Practice nurses have physical health care skills but lack training and confidence to implement these effectively with people with serious mental illness (Lester et al., 2005). The design of health services, which separates physical and mental health care and requires collaboration and communication across differently funded service interfaces, contributes to a system where individual needs cannot easily be met. This is despite the UK government's support for a holistic approach to care or 'parity of esteem' (Royal College of Psychiatrists, 2013).

# THE SERIOUS MENTAL ILLNESS HEALTH IMPROVEMENT PROFILE (HIP)

The Health Improvement Profile (HIP) was designed as a practical way to help mental health nurses profile the physical health of the people with serious mental illness whom they work with. The aim was to help the nurse complete a health check to identify any physical health parameters outside their 'normal' range and work together with the service user to agree the best action to take next. The parameters identified in the HIP are those considered most at risk in people with a serious mental illness diagnosis (see Table 10.1). There are male and female versions of the HIP because a few of the parameter ranges are gender specific (menstrual cycle, for example). The HIP is evidence-based because the included items, their individual ranges and next steps are based on recommendations from published research, expert consensus and/or health policy (White et al., 2009; White, 2015).

**Table 10.1  Physical health parameters at risk in serious mental illness that are included in the Health Improvement Profile (HIP)**

| | | | |
|---|---|---|---|
| 1. | Body Mass Index (BMI) | 15. | Breast check (female and male) |
| 2. | Waist circumference | 16. | Menstrual cycle (female) |
| 3. | Pulse | 17. | Smoking status |
| 4. | Blood Pressure | 18. | Exercise |
| 5. | Temperature | 19. | Alcohol intake |
| 6. | Liver Function Tests | 20. | Diet: 5-a-day |
| 7. | Lipid levels | 21. | Diet: fat intake |
| 8. | Glucose | 22. | Fluid intake |
| 9. | Cervical smear (female) | 23. | Caffeine intake |
| 10. | Prostate and testicles check (male) | 24. | Cannabis use |
| 11. | Sleep | 25. | Safe sex |
| 12. | Teeth | 26. | Urine |
| 13. | Eyes | 27. | Bowels |
| 14. | Feet | 28. | Sexual satisfaction |

> ### ⚙ REFLECTION POINT 10.2
>
> - Take a few minutes to reflect on your own physical health skills.
> - Do you think that you can accurately measure blood pressure, identify whether the result is abnormal and know what to do if it is too low or too high?
> - What would you say to a service user who complains of feeling tired and lacking in energy all day? What other information would you want from them? Would you undertake or refer them for any tests? What information would you exchange with them about what they can do to try to change how they are feeling?
> - If your answer to any of the above is 'no' or 'not sure', what can you do to change this?

## USING THE HIP

The HIP is intended to be completed on an annual basis, which is the recommended frequency of screening for individuals with serious mental illness in England (NICE, 2014a: CG7.2.8.5). As authors of the HIP, we believed that it was important that it was not used as a checklist for assessment but that it prompted evidence-based action for any parameters that were identified to be at risk. The HIP was therefore designed to direct the nurse to work with the service user to select the action or actions to take next that best suited them by providing a menu of possible interventions to choose from. Citations were provided for all parameter ranges and recommended actions. Where there was the potential of different tests being used in practice (for example, for blood glucose), a range of alternatives were included.

The original HIP was designed to fit on one side of a sheet of paper so that mental health nurses in practice could easily copy and use it. It was believed that a paper-based version would be more readily adopted and could easily be photocopied and sent to the service user's GP or other agency, with a cover letter to provide supporting evidence for any recommended referral.

The HIP has columns indicating the variable at risk for assessment (for example, smoking status), level (result), Green (for example, 'non-smoker'), Red (for example, 'passive smoker/smoker') and the recommended action for the Red group (for example, advice that all smoking is associated with health risks, refer to NHS smoking cessation service). For a second example, BMI, see Table 10.2.

There was a need to consider issues of intellectual property against motivation to disseminate the HIP as widely as possible and encourage its implementation. A paper describing the development of the HIP and its initial dissemination was published in the leading journal for mental health nursing in the UK (White et al., 2009). A copy of the HIP was not included in the publication but was released to anyone who made contact with us and agreed to provide feedback in future via email. This dissemination work continues today and the ongoing dialogue with the large network of users is helpful in regularly updating the HIP. For example, in

**Table 10.2    The Body Mass Index (BMI) parameter**

| Parameter | Level | Green | Red | Recommended action for red group |
|---|---|---|---|---|
| BMI | | 18.50–24.99[1] | <18.50[1] | • BMI, 18.50 – refer for further investigations |
| | | | ≥ 25.00*[1] | • BMI ≥ 25.00 – advice and support on diet and exercise, referral to local weight/exercise management programme, consider medication review[2] |

*Notes:* [1] WHO (2007). This is the BMI for Europids, please refer to ethnic-specific values where required.

[2] Barnett et al. (2007).

* Overweight = BMI > 23.00 in individuals of South Asian origin.

2012, changes were made to the blood pressure parameter and, in 2014, to the diet parameters, due to new published guidance and feedback from users. The UK version of the HIP and the *Health Improvement Profile Manual* have since been published (Hardy et al., 2015).

A flexible training package was prepared that could be delivered in a 1–4 hour workshop to enable those attending to understand how to:

1. Use the HIP and the *Health Improvement Profile Manual* to systematically examine the physical health of individual service users and identify the best next steps to take for items that flag Red.
2. Use the results to agree an individual health action plan.
3. Identify barriers and levers to implementation and construct an action plan to support the use of the HIP in practice.

Mental health nurses consistently report a positive attitude towards physical health care as part of their role in working with people with serious mental illness, but state that they require training to enable them to enact the role. Their perception of low baseline knowledge to inform physical health care practice in serious mental illness was confirmed and significant knowledge gain immediately after the HIP training demonstrated in 38 mental health nurses via a pre- and post-training evaluation (White et al., 2014).

---

⚙ **REFLECTION POINT 10.3**

- Consider each of the parameters in Table 10.1. Make a note of any of them that you feel you lack enough knowledge, skills or confidence to start to address with the service users whom you encounter in your practice.
- For each of the items on your list, consider using a problem-solving approach to identify SMART* goals to address them.

*SMART = Specific, Measurable, Acceptable, Realistic and Time limited

# EVIDENCE FROM IMPLEMENTATION OF THE HIP

Early pilot work demonstrated that the HIP can be used in clinical practice and was acceptable to service users, nurses, psychiatrists and GPs (Shuel et al., 2010; White, 2010). Practice nurses were successfully trained to use the primary care version (Hardy and Gray, 2010; Hardy et al., 2014). Electronic record systems are more usual in mental health services than when the HIP was first developed and many organisations have constructed electronic versions of the HIP to support standardised care pathways, clinical audit and reporting of data to commissioners. These 'eHIP' versions often include additional 'amber' ranges that indicate more frequent (than annual) monitoring when results are at the upper or lower ranges of normal. Some organisations have phased implementation of the HIP, so that metabolic parameters are prioritised within the first two weeks of an (acute) admission and other parameters addressed later in the care pathway.

The HIP has been used to screen thousands of service users with serious mental illness from across the UK, and is the focus of local Commissioning for Quality and Innovation (CQUIN) targets in six UK mental health provider organisations. Academics from 12 countries worldwide have accessed the HIP to adapt it for their serious mental illness populations. There are US, Swiss, German, Chinese and Thai versions and there is a growing body of literature that describes the health profile of people with serious mental illness where the HIP is being used, and some evidence that health outcomes are improved where it is used in the same person over time (Bressington et al., 2013, 2014, 2016; Bänziger et al., 2016; Thongsai et al., 2016).

How best to implement health screening to improve health and quality of life outcomes in people with serious mental illness who access care from community mental health services remains a significant challenge. A cluster randomised controlled trial of the HIP demonstrated that the process of using the HIP by community mental health nurses in routine practice in the UK after training did not improve service users' health-related quality of life over a year (White, 2015). The trial took place against a background of significant reconfiguration of community services across all study sites, including the decommissioning of assertive outreach teams. Of the community mental health nurses in the trial who were randomised to the HIP training, only 42% completed the HIP with their consented study participants at baseline and only 28% at a year, considerably weakening any inferences that could be drawn about effectiveness. A process observation that included interviews and a case note audit took place immediately after the trial in a subsample of the HIP group participants. This demonstrated that, despite service users expressing a wish for their community mental health nurses to undertake physical health care, nurses experienced barriers related to clinical engagement and organisation of their work. These barriers were reported to impact on their ability to intervene beyond assessment and/or repeat the HIP at a year. These findings are not unusual to the HIP as a study that used the Rethink Physical Health Check (Phelan et al., 2004) also identified implementation barriers by (community) care coordinators (National Institute for Health Research, Collaboration for Leadership in Applied Health Research and Care, (CLAHRC) for Greater Manchester, 2013).

Studies to investigate the experiences of community mental health nurses who have used the HIP in the UK and Hong Kong provide some insight into the facilitators and barriers to its successful use in practice (White, 2015; Bressington et al., 2016). The opportunity to work systematically and comprehensively with service user physical health needs was welcomed by both groups of nurses who reported how the HIP helped them refocus attention on physical issues and holistic care needs. Profiling using the HIP made sure that important issues that were not routinely assessed or raised by service users were the subject of a structured enquiry (for example, sexual health). Use of the HIP also highlighted training needs, specifically to help the mental health nurses have more confidence when discussing the potential consequences of parameters that were outside the normal range (or any subsequent diagnosis, for example hyperlipidaemia). Service-level barriers were identified that highlighted a need for more integrated care. This included (in both groups) the identification of cultural barriers to communication and agreement between different disciplines that impacted negatively on multidisciplinary working (for example, between community mental health nurses and GPs, between psychiatrists and GPs). A perception of a move towards a more acute service in mental health provision as a consequence of austerity was reported by the UK community mental health nurses as a barrier to working long enough with individuals to engage them in annual health screening and intervention, particularly those interventions designed to effect health behaviour change over time (White, 2015). Nurses in both countries described a lack of services they could refer service users to for specific interventions (for example, weight management).

There is the potential to address these issues through an integrated process of commissioning around the needs of the population of people with serious mental illness, rather than the commissioning of specific services to meet specific needs. Where the HIP has been commissioned as part of a CQUIN, it has been implemented, although care has also been needed to make sure that recording of data for audit purposes in an electronic record has not become an administrative exercise removed from the service user. It is important that the HIP results inform what was intended, a joint discussion between mental health nurses and service users about their physical health needs and an agreed plan about what to do next to start to address these.

## ACTIVITY 10.1   PERSONAL AND PROFESSIONAL ACTION PLAN

Revisit the list of SMART goals made in the last exercise. Consider if additional service or systems level goals may be required. Identify who you can talk to about these and arrange to have a conversation with them. How do mental health nurses who want to develop and/or maintain their physical health care knowledge and skills after registration access support and supervision?

## CONCLUSION

The serious mental illness Health Improvement Profile was developed as a pragmatic assessment to target physical wellbeing in people with serious mental illness through the existing role of the mental health nurses in secondary care. It was intended to support mental health nurses working with people with serious mental illness to undertake a structured health check and negotiate and implement an individualised physical health care plan. There is good evidence of clinical utility of the HIP and a growing body of evidence of an improvement in health outcomes where it has been used as intended to support health checks and intervention in the same person over time. The HIP is well liked by clinicians and service users and there is no evidence of any harm from its use. It continues to be used across the UK and internationally by nurses, services and commissioners of mental health services. How best to design services and care pathways so that people with serious mental illness living in the community can have their physical health needs met remains a significant challenge. Studies suggest that more work is needed to commission and develop integrated care pathways and services that will enable the aspirations of holistic care to become reality.

## USEFUL RESOURCES

Hardy, S. and Gray, R. (2012) *The Primary Care Guide to Mental Health*. Keswick: M&K Publishing.

An uncomplicated guide to the range of mental health problems seen in primary care. From common mental health problems like depression to rare conditions like schizophrenia, this resource provides the background needed to help students and clinicians understand care and treatment options.

Hardy, S., White, J. and Gray, R. (2015) *The Health Improvement Profile: A Manual to Promote Physical Wellbeing in People with Severe Mental Illness*. Keswick: M&K Publishing.

An introduction to physical comorbidities and problematic health behaviours in serious mental illness. Explains how to use the Health Improvement Profile to screen, inrevene and help people with serious mental illness change their health behaviour. Includes copies of the male and female HIP.

Royal College of Psychiatrists web page. Improving Mental and Physical Health. Available at: www.rcpsych.ac.uk/mentalhealthinfo/improvingphysicalandmh.aspx (accessed 3 October 2016).

Provides links to a range of recommended resources to support physical health care in people with mental illness and to support mental health care in people with physical illness.

## ANSWERS TO MULTIPLE CHOICE QUESTIONS

1(b), 2(d), 3(c), 4(a), 5(a), 6(d), 7(c), 8(d), 9(b), 10(c)

# OVERCOMING COMMON BARRIERS TO HEALTH AND WELLBEING

# PART THREE

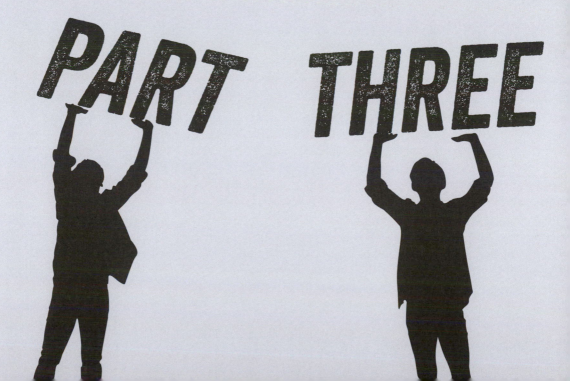

# ELEVEN

## ACTIVATION FOR PHYSICAL AND MENTAL WELLBEING

### HILARY MAIRS

### CHAPTER LEARNING OUTCOMES

After reading this chapter, you will be able to:

- Describe a behavioural activation approach to promote both physical and mental health.
- Outline the extant evidence base and theoretical underpinning for this approach.
- Discuss the relevance of behavioural activation for the service users with whom you work.

## MULTIPLE CHOICE QUESTIONS

We have included 10 multiple choice questions at the beginning of this chapter for readers wishing to test their knowledge of its contents. We have included the answers at the end of the chapter, but advise you not to check these until you have answered them before and after reading the chapter so that you can determine how much your knowledge has increased.

1. Goals work best when they are:

    a) Aligned to service targets.
    b) Set retrospectively.
    c) Specific, Measurable, Acceptable, Realistic and Time (SMART)-limited.
    d) Written in the third person.

2. Behavioural activation involves:

    a) Scheduling pleasant activities only.
    b) Helping people to think about themselves differently.
    c) Taking a full developmental history from the service user about the causes of the problem.
    d) Graded activation in line with individual goals and values.

*(Continued)*

*(Continued)*

3. The evidence for behavioural activation at the present time is:

   a)  Largely based on small studies of limited methodological quality.
   b)  Best established for anxiety problems.
   c)  Strong enough for policy-makers in the UK to recommend it as a first-line treatment for depression.
   d)  Based on a substantial number of cohort studies with long-term outcomes.

4. Setting an agenda at the start of each session ensures that:

   a)  Sessions can be relatively short.
   b)  The practitioner can lead on the content of the session.
   c)  Time can be used efficiently to focus on behavioural activation.
   d)  There is plenty of time to discuss the origins of their mental health problem.

5. The concept of an activity hierarchy is borrowed from:

   a)  Psychoanalytic psychotherapy.
   b)  Graded exposure treatments for anxiety problems.
   c)  Non-directive counselling.
   d)  Group therapies.

6. Strategies to enhance the likelihood that a person will complete a between-session activation task include:

   a)  A clear rationale for the task and discussion about any predicted obstacles.
   b)  The involvement of significant others.
   c)  The detail of the task being decided on by the mental health practitioner.
   d)  Using the same task each time.

7. Positive reinforcement:

   a)  Involves the addition of something that an individual finds rewarding and/or pleasurable after a specific behaviour that increases the likelihood that the behaviour will be repeated.
   b)  Always comprises significant financial reward.
   c)  Includes removing something unpleasant after a behaviour.
   d)  Is the sole focus of behavioural activation.

8. One of the benefits of behavioural activation is that:

   a)  It is relatively straightforward and may require less staff training.
   b)  It is a well-established treatment for a number of mental and physical health problems.
   c)  There is overwhelming evidence that service users find the approach acceptable.
   d)  It was developed some ago.

9. Friends and family of people who want to increase their activity levels:

   a)  Should always be involved in the process.
   b)  Should always be excluded from the process.
   c)  May be included if this is considered to be helpful on an individual basis.
   d)  None of the above.

10. The behavioural activation process:

   a) Requires that all six stages are followed in a linear way.
   b) Should be used flexibly to ensure that the service user remains engaged in the approach.
   c) Requires significant training on the part of the practitioner.
   d) Is not well established.


# INTRODUCTION

This chapter will outline an approach called 'behavioural activation', which was originally devised as a treatment for depression but is now much more widely applied to address a number of mental health and related physical health problems. This relatively parsimonious (straightforward) intervention aims to help people re-establish the weekly routines that will promote both mental and physical wellbeing by increasing their activity levels in line with their own aspirations, values and goals. The approach is underpinned by an emerging evidence base and behavioural theories of reinforcement (which we will explain in further detail below). It is an individualised intervention that acknowledges that retreat and reduced levels of activity are often a way of coping with mental health problems (or the problems that led to the onset of this) and that this can be protective in the short term. However, if left unchecked, reduced levels of activity are often associated with a worsening of the mental health problem and an increased risk of poor physical health. In Chapter 7, we discussed the low levels of physical activity that are associated with a range of different mental health problems. We have also acknowledged the link between inactivity and smoking (Chapter 8).

Behavioural activation is a staged approach and it can be helpful to think of it as being based on six individual phases. Although, in practice, it is rare that these six stages are followed in a linear way, they are presented here in this way for the purposes of clarity. The six stages are:

1. Activity monitoring
2. Values and activity identification
3. Activity ranking
4. Goal-setting;
5. Goal implementation
6. Activity review.

The behavioural activation approach described here is based on the versions designed for depression and tested by Lejuez et al. (2011) in the USA and Richards and Whyte (2011) in the UK.

# THE THEORY UNDERPINNING BEHAVIOURAL ACTIVATION

The earliest behavioural activation treatments were described in the 1970s, and were based on the theory proposed by Lewinsohn and Graf (1973) that the environmental stressors that contribute to the development of depression are associated with reduced levels of positive reinforcement in combination with a limited range of interpersonal skills.

Some readers will be familiar with behavioural theories of reinforcement but for those who are not we provide a brief explanation here. These theories suggest that we are much more likely to repeat behaviours when they are reinforced in some way. Positive reinforcement involves the addition of something that an individual finds rewarding and/or pleasurable. This favourable outcome, reward or event after the behaviour increases the likelihood that it will be repeated. For example, a shy person who goes to a party and makes a number of friends with whom they have shared interests is more likely to go a party again in the future. In contrast, negative reinforcement involves the removal of something that an individual finds unpleasant or stressful which also increases the likelihood that the behaviour will be repeated. A commonly cited example of negative reinforcement focuses on someone with chronic pain who may go back to bed because, previously, this led to a reduction in pain levels (Kanter et al., 2009).

---

⚙️  **REFLECTION POINT 11.1**

Think about activities in your own life such as playing sport, cooking, gardening, dancing, etc. that you are more likely to participate in because you have received positive reinforcement from those around you. Supposing that you hadn't received positive reinforcement, how might it have affected your behaviour?

---

The earliest descriptions of behavioural activation focused on the scheduling of activities designed to increase exposure to a range of positive reinforcement. Later accounts have highlighted the additional role played by negative reinforcement, noting that the reduced level of activity observed in depression is often maintained because of withdrawal and avoidance of activities that an individual needs to do. Hence, the focus of contemporary behavioural activation approaches is identifying 'depressed behaviours' and developing alternative goal-orientated behaviours that address avoidance (Rhodes et al., 2014).

As we have already highlighted, the original behavioural activation approaches were tested as treatments for depression, but more recently they have been adapted and tested for other mental health and the related physical health problems that we have already discussed in this book. The following review in no way constitutes a systematic review but provides an overview of some of the evidence for behavioural activation in addressing complex mental and physical health problems.

## BEHAVIOURAL ACTIVATION FOR MENTAL HEALTH PROBLEMS

As noted above, behavioural activation was originally devised as a treatment for depression and a number of studies have found that behavioural activation is an effective remedy for low mood (Ekers et al., 2008). Unfortunately, the methodological quality of these studies has often been limited and, consequently, the National Institute for Health and Care Excellence (NICE) in the UK does not recommend it at present as a first-line treatment for depression (NICE, 2009: CG90). However, they do recommend further research to determine whether behavioural activation is an effective alternative to cognitive behavioural therapy (which they recommend for depression) and, indeed, a study is underway to compare these two treatments in a robust randomised controlled trial (Rhodes et al., 2014). The criticisms of the behavioural activation for depression evidence base also applies for other mental health problems. Many studies suggest that behavioural activation is a promising treatment for post-traumatic stress (Jakupcak et al., 2010) and psychosis (Mairs et al., 2011; Waller et al., 2013). Further research is underway to establish whether behavioural activation may be an effective alternative to more complex therapies for a range of mental health problems. It is also useful to note that behavioural activation is often used as a component of cognitive behavioural therapy, the psychological treatment of choice for a number of mental health problems.

## BEHAVIOURAL ACTIVATION FOR OBESITY

In an initial investigation, Pagoto et al. (2008) developed a behavioural activation treatment protocol to emphasise excessive eating as a depressive behaviour and participants were encouraged to schedule activities promoting enjoyment and achievement which were: (1) incompatible with eating; and (2) increased levels of physical activity. In addition to this adapted form of behavioural activation, participants also received six group sessions focusing on diet counselling. Results of this uncontrolled evaluation suggest that the intervention was feasible and acceptable and, further, that it led to reductions in weight and caloric intake as well as increases in physical activity. At the same time, significant reductions in depression were also observed. However, in a more robust, sufficiently powered randomised controlled trial (Pagoto et al., 2013), no differences in weight loss, changes in daily energy intake or daily physical activity were found between those in receipt of behavioural activation and those who instead received the control lifestyle intervention. However, there were significant differences in levels of depression observed between the two groups at both 6 and 12 months post-intervention, with those in the behavioural activation condition showing significantly greater reductions in depression.

In a later study, Alfonsson et al. (2015) evaluated a group behavioural activation treatment for people with severe obesity and binge eating disorder (BED). The group behavioural activation treatment consisted of 10 sessions and included the following components: psycho-education, planned activation, identification of avoidance behaviours, thought-action diffusion, problem-solving, social activation and goal-setting. Consistent with the controlled trial discussed above, those in the behavioural activation group reported significantly lower levels of depression, but there were no differences between the behavioural activation group and those in the waiting list control group in terms of weight loss.

Both Pagoto et al. (2013) and Alfonsson et al. (2015) suggest that further attention to behavioural patterns that maintain problem eating as well as attention to the behaviours that maintain depression may be required to demonstrate an impact on eating patterns and weight gain; although at the time of writing this chapter, no evaluations of these adapted treatments had been reported, so it is unclear whether such changes to behavioural activation protocols would ensure that they were more effective in addressing weight gain or not.

## BEHAVIOURAL ACTIVATION TO AID SMOKING CESSATION

MacPherson et al. (2010) conducted a randomised controlled trial of an 8-session behavioural activation smoking cessation treatment for smokers with elevated depressive symptoms. In their study, the behavioural activation treatment was associated with reductions in both smoking and depression, although these findings need to be interpreted with some caution because of a number of factors related to the design of the study, for example the use of a treatment as usual control group and the high number of people who refused to take part in the study.

Further research into the effectiveness of behavioural activation is clearly required and is underway. These developments are driven, at least in part, by the fact the behavioural activation rationale is relatively simple and potentially straightforward to operationalise for both mental health practitioners and service users (Rhodes et al., 2014).

### KEY MESSAGE 11.1

- There is an emerging evidence base that suggests that behavioural activation may be an effective treatment for helping people with both mental and physical health issues.
- If shown to be successful in these trials, behavioural activation may be a more straightforward and therefore less expensive alternative to more traditional therapies such as cognitive behavioural therapy.

# THE RATIONALE FOR BEHAVIOURAL ACTIVATION

As we highlighted in the introduction to this chapter, there are six stages to a behavioural activation approach and we will describe each of these in turn. As with other psychosocial and psychological treatments, it is vital that the service user is provided with a clear rationale for behavioural activation so that they can make an informed decision as to whether they wish to participate in the approach; that is, they agree with the mental health practitioner that this is the optimal approach to attempt at this time. This is likely to strengthen the therapeutic alliance (Bordin, 1979): the quality of the relationship between the practitioner and the service user. One of the other benefits of the rationale that we have found helpful is that it normalises the reduced levels of activity observed in many mental health problems. The rationale is likely to include some of the points listed in Key Message 11.2.

## KEY MESSAGE 11.2

- Reduced levels of activity are common when people have mental health problems and this can be a useful way of coping in the initial stages, however remaining inactive is likely to contribute further to mental health problems as well as physical health problems.
- Increasing activity in a graded way when the time seems right for the service user (rather than for other people) can be helpful.
- The process requires the active engagement of the service user in the process because much of the work will be done outside of the formal behavioural activation sessions.

## THE STRUCTURE OF BEHAVIOURAL ACTIVATION

Behavioural activation, like other psychosocial and psychological therapies, benefits from being facilitated in a structured way. Adopting a structured approach can help to promote the active engagement that will be required if increases in activity levels are to be realised. Scheduling sessions at the same time each week, month or fortnight can help a person to re-establish the routine that will support activation. Setting an agenda at the beginning of each session can help to keep an important focus on behavioural activation and ensure that the time is used productively. Providing regular summaries and requesting feedback about the process can help to mark the collaboration required if the service user is to engage fully in the process. Ultimately, the success of the approach will be down to the extent to which the service user engages in the activation exercises between sessions and a sound individual rationale to the approach and well-structured sessions will facilitate this (Mairs, 2017).

## THE FIRST STAGE: COMPLETING AN ACTIVITY DIARY OR SCHEDULE

The first stage of the process requires finding out about what the service user is currently doing on a day-to-day basis by charting the detail of their weekly routine. This is commonly achieved via the completion of an activity diary or schedule such as the one in Table 11.1, usually as homework or a between-session task. The reasons for advising that it is done in this way include that this is the optimal way to capture accurately what the service user is doing by recording this as close to real time as possible, and also that it introduces the idea that participation in exercises between treatment sessions (sometimes referred to as 'homework') is key to the success of the approach. A completed diary then provides a clear picture of how a person is spending their time, although some approaches recommend that additional information such as mood ratings or levels of enjoyment and achievement are also recorded.

**Table 11.1   An example of an activity diary**

|           | Sun | Mon | Tues | Wed | Thurs | Fri | Sat |
|-----------|-----|-----|------|-----|-------|-----|-----|
| Morning   |     |     |      |     |       |     |     |
| Afternoon |     |     |      |     |       |     |     |
| Evening   |     |     |      |     |       |     |     |

There are a number of strategies that will enhance the likelihood that the task will be completed successfully. First, it is vital to give a clear and individual rationale for the value of completing the diary or schedule. Second, it is important to spend some time within the session completing a part of the diary so that the service user has chance to practise this before attempting to do so without the support of the practitioner. Third, it is useful to ask whether the service user can identify any obstacles that may prevent them from completing the diary and then spend some time problem solving any such barriers to successful completion of the homework task. Creative solutions may be required where people struggle with writing things down, are worried that they may forget or find it difficult to see the point of completing an activity diary.

The best activity diaries and schedules are those that have been devised individually and chart for each individual the information that they and the practitioner will find most useful. Some schedules allow for the recording of activities on an hour-by-hour basis, but this might be too onerous for someone with a complex mental health problem. Once a diary has been completed, it is important to review the schedule and determine whether a person is satisfied with how they are spending their time or whether they would like to make changes to their activity levels and engage in the next stage of the process.

## THE SECOND STAGE: VALUES AND ACTIVITY IDENTIFICATION

The second stage of the process focuses on generating a list of activities that the service user would like to do more often or to begin to introduce into their weekly routine. In line with the behavioural theory on which the treatment is based, the activities selected should increase access to positive reinforcement and address any avoidance. To this end, Richards and Whyte (2011) have advised that the list should include a mix of pleasurable, necessary and routine activities. Including a focus on necessary activities ensures that the importance of addressing avoidance is not forgotten. It can also be helpful to include a number of activities that necessitate contact with other people. Some service users may readily identify the activities that will help them to meet this aim but for others this may be more difficult. Where this is the case, it can be useful to spend some time helping people to identify their values as a first stage to selecting pleasurable, necessary and routine activities (Lejuez et al., 2011).

Values have been described as desired global qualities of ongoing action: indicating the direction in which a person wants to move, where goals and activities are, what they would need to achieve along the way (Kanter et al., 2009). The concept is often illustrated by way of considering the value of heading west. Activities might include the climbing of a mountain or crossing of a river while travelling west. A more concrete example is someone who holds the value of being a loving parent and identifies that the following activities would indicate that they are travelling in the direction of being a loving parent; they might decide to tell their children that they love them every day, make a special effort to cook one of their favourite meals for them at the weekend or ensure that they meet them at the school gates promptly each week day (Lejuez et al., 2011). The concept of values is borrowed from a related psychotherapy called Acceptance and Commitment Therapy (ACT) and a number of resources are available to help practitioners and service users identify their values as a first stage of selecting activities that will help them to move in this direction and access diverse, stable and valued sources of reinforcement along the way (ibid.). The Brief Behavioural Activation Treatment for Depression treatment manual advises considering values in a number of different life areas or domains, relationships, education/occupation, recreation/interests, mind/body/spirituality and daily activities (ibid.).

**ii̇̇ni̇̇   CASE STUDY 11.1**

Azera identified a value to finding meaningful employment. It was less important that she was paid for any work she did than that she found something to do that fitted well with her skills and interests. With her mental health practitioner, she generated a list of activities that would facilitate her moving in the direction of securing a job, which included talking to the employment worker within the mental health team and looking through the local job opportunities online.

**✿̇̇   REFLECTION POINT 11.2**

Generate a list of activities that would support a person wishing to move in line with the following values:

- To be a respected member of the community.
- To be physically healthy.
- To be a compassionate manager.

An additional benefit of thinking about values is that it shifts to a constructive focus from the problem of what someone is not doing to thinking about what they would like to be doing.

## THE THIRD STAGE: GENERATING AN ACTIVITY HIERARCHY

In the third stage, the selected activities are ranked according to the perceived level of difficulty in an activity hierarchy, in much the same way that activities are ranked in a hierarchy to inform a graded exposure treatment for agoraphobia. It has been suggested that ranking no more than 12 activities that include a sound mix of pleasurable, necessary and routine activities is a solid basis for an activity hierarchy (Richards and Whyte, 2011). It is critical to be mindful that it is the service user's perception of difficulty that should guide where individual activities are ranked within the hierarchy and also that some modification in the ordering of activities may be required from time to time.

## THE FOURTH STAGE: ACTIVITY PLANNING AND SCHEDULING

In the fourth stage of the behavioural activation process, goals are set to help service users gradually introduce the activities ranked in the previous stage into their weekly routine. The aim is to begin working at bottom and work systemically up the activity hierarchy in order to increase activity in a graded way and maximise the likelihood of success. We know that in a number of mental health conditions people develop unhelpful beliefs about their own abilities to be successful or to enjoy participating in activities, either because of the experiences that contributed to the development of the mental health problem (Rector, 2014) or because they change the way in which they think about their own abilities as a result of having become depressed or developing psychosis (Staring et al., 2013). Consequently, it is important to avoid reinforcing these beliefs by setting goals that are unachievable.

It is therefore important that the goals that are set are SMART – that is: Specific, Measurable, Acceptable, Realistic and Time limited – although we will later on discuss the benefits of working with SMARTER goals. This is because SMART goals work best (Simmons and Griffiths, 2014), and ensure that it is clear what will be done, by whom and when. It is also important that the goals reflect the aspirations of the service user, rather than those of other people. We have learned from clinical experience that goals which are more aligned to the service provider rather than the individual service user's ambitions are unlikely to be realised.

Goal-setting, like other skills, requires practice and those of you less familiar with the process may wish to practise your goal-setting skills in the exercise in Reflection Point 11.3.

---

## ⚙ REFLECTION POINT 11.3

Rework the following goals so that they conform to the SMART criteria as far as is possible without an in-depth knowledge of the people setting the goals:

- Abdul will get up early on three occasions.
- Rukshar will increase her activity levels by cycling each week for a month.
- Rachel will join a gym.

---

We recommend that the following process is adopted when setting goals as part of a behavioural activation process. Where activities have been generated after the identification of individual values, it can be helpful to note the specific value guiding the selection of the activity before setting a SMART goal to inform the who, what, where and when the activity will be implemented. Recording this in an activity schedule or record is key. We have included an example from one of Azera's activity diaries below in Table 11.2. It can also be motivating to assess the benefits or positive outcomes of achieving the goal, and important to consider whether there are predictable barriers or obstacles that need to be problem-solved to maximise the likelihood of goal attainment. It has also been suggested that goals are more likely to be achieved if the detail of the activity is shared with at least one other person.

**Table 11.2  An example of Azera's activity schedule**

|  | Sun | Mon | Tues | Wed | Thurs | Fri | Sat |
|---|---|---|---|---|---|---|---|
| **Morning** |  | Make an appointment to meet with employment contact |  |  |  |  |  |
| **Afternoon** |  |  |  | Spend 30 minutes looking at local jobs online and making a note of any that seem possibilities |  |  |  |
| **Evening** |  |  |  |  |  |  |  |

## THE FIFTH STAGE: ACTIVITY IMPLEMENTATION

Successful engagement with the behavioural activation approach will require that much of the work done takes place between sessions. Hence, the importance of paying particular attention to the setting of goals in the stage discussed above. In the early stages of this process, behavioural activation sessions may be fairly regular but, as a service user becomes engaged in the approach, it may be helpful to space sessions out so that there is more time for them to complete the activation exercises. It is still important to schedule sessions though to provide feedback and trouble-shoot any difficulties that arise during the process. The spacing-out of sessions also reinforces the idea that behavioural activation is a time-limited treatment and that, at some point, the practitioner and service user will begin to plan for the end of the intervention.

## THE SIXTH STAGE: ACTIVITY REVIEW

This stage focuses on the within-session review of the implementation of activity and goal attainment, the ER of SMARTER goals: Evaluation and Review. Where goals have been met, it is important that the practitioner provides positive feedback (which can be reinforcing in and of itself) and helps the service user begin to think about the next stage of the process, which will usually be to set goals in relation to activities higher up the activity hierarchy.

Where goals have not been met, it is critical to praise any attempts to achieve the goal and troubleshoot the reasons why the goal was not attained. Where this was due to unforeseen circumstances, such as someone having a heavy cold, the goal may be rescheduled for the following week. However, if the practitioner and service user decide that the goal is unrealistic at the present time, they should work together to reformulate the goal and set a more achievable one. It can sometimes be helpful for the practitioner to take responsibility for not making the goal clear enough, for example, in order to avoid reinforcing any unhelpful defeatist beliefs that the service user may hold about their abilities to succeed and/or enjoy.

## FRIENDS, FAMILY AND COMPANIONS

The extent to which it can be helpful to involve other people in a behavioural activation approach is likely to vary from person to person. For some people, it may be really helpful, in the short term at least, to involve friends and families in their activation exercises. However, for other people, it may actually be counter-productive, particularly where friends and families expect people to make progress more quickly than they are able to do (Mairs et al., 2012). Hence, deciding when and how to involve other people will need to be determined on an individual basis.

## CHALLENGES IN IMPLEMENTING A BEHAVIOURAL ACTIVATION APPROACH

We have already highlighted the importance of working with a service user at the time that is right for them. In the instance that a service user is ambivalent about increasing their activity levels, it can sometimes be helpful to engage them in a process of decisional balance, exploring the advantages of becoming more active and the disadvantages of not doing so (Chapter 12). Charting these advantages and disadvantages on a sheet of paper such as the one presented in Table 11.3 can be beneficial. Where advantages outweigh disadvantages, it can also be helpful to record the three most important reasons for a person to increase their activity levels to enhance motivation throughout the behavioural activation process.

For some people, the main barrier to engaging in a behavioural activation approach may be the defeatist beliefs they hold about their own abilities to complete everyday tasks, enjoy the activities that they used to and/or make meaningful relationships (Mairs, 2017). Where this is the case, helping people explore these beliefs in further detail in a process called 'cognitive restructuring' may be required. Such approaches often include behavioural experiments

**Table 11.3   An example of a decisional balance record sheet**

|  | Becoming more active | Not becoming more active |
|---|---|---|
| Advantages |  |  |
| Disadvantages |  |  |
| Three reasons to become more active:<br>1.<br>2.<br>3. |  |  |

that are designed to help people test out how accurate their predictions are as a way of generating evidence to counteract these negative defeatist beliefs (Westbrook et al., 2011).

# THE PROCESS OF BEHAVIOURAL ACTIVATION

We have already recommended that behavioural activation sessions are scheduled at regular intervals and that sessions may become more spaced out over time, once service users have become proficient in setting their own goals. This also communicates a message that the behavioural activation process is a time-limited one. In order to ensure that any gains are maintained at the end of the intervention, it can be helpful for the practitioner and service user to spend some time in later sessions drafting a summary of what has been learnt and developing an action plan as to what they will do if they notice that they are becoming less active and beginning to avoid their normal day-to-day activities.

> ## ⚙ REFLECTION POINT 11.4
>
> Think about the service users with whom you are working at the moment and whether there are any of them whom you think might benefit from participating in the structured behavioural activation approach that we outlined here. Can you think of any obstacles that you may experience in engaging them in this way of working and any possible strategies to overcome these barriers?

## CONCLUSION

Behavioural activation is a structured, parsimonious treatment that offers promise in promoting both the mental and physical health for people with complex mental health needs. It is based on a normalising premise that withdrawing from stress can be protective in the short term, while acknowledging the problems that long-term avoidance brings in relation to mental and physical wellbeing. It is a key point that the goals set reflect service user rather than service values and that activation is paced according to individual need. Decisions to engage others in the process need to be carefully considered to determine whether any potential costs outweigh the benefits.

## USEFUL RESOURCES

Mairs, H. (2017) *Revisiting Negative Symptoms: Working with Reduced Expression and Activity in Psychosis*. London: Palgrave Macmillan.

This book provides an overview of behavioural activation and other approaches to help people with psychosis who have become inactive. It is a highly practical and accessible guide for practitioners who regularly work with this group of service users.

Richards, D.A. and Whyte, M. (2011) *Reach Out: National Programme Educator Materials to Support the Delivery of Psychological Wellbeing Practitioners Delivering Low-Intensity Interventions*, 3rd edn. London: Rethink.

This publication provides details on how to facilitate behavioural activation for people with the common mental health problems of anxiety and depression.

## ANSWERS TO MULTIPLE CHOICE QUESTIONS

1(c), 2(d), 3(a), 4(c), 5(b), 6(a), 7(a), 8(a), 9(c), 10(b)

# TWELVE

## MOTIVATIONAL INTERVIEWING FOR POSITIVE LIFESTYLE CHOICES

### IAN WILSON

## CHAPTER LEARNING OUTCOMES

After reading this chapter, you will be able to:

- Describe what motivational interviewing is.
- Understand its historical development and its evolution as a way of talking to people about change.
- Be aware of the evidence base that underpins motivational interviewing.
- Consider the principles of motivational interviewing and its core skills, and understand the 'spirit' that underpins them.
- Begin to see how these skills can be applied when working with the physical health problems experienced by people with mental health problems.

## MULTIPLE CHOICE QUESTIONS

We have included 10 multiple choice questions at the beginning of this chapter for readers wishing to test their knowledge of its contents. We have included the answers at the end of the chapter, but advise you not to check these until you have answered them before and after reading the chapter so that you can determine how much your knowledge has increased.

1. Motivational interviewing is used when talking to people about potential change in:

    a) Alcohol and drug misuse.
    b) Tobacco smoking.
    c) Diet and exercise.
    d) All of the above.

2. The efficacy of motivational interviewing has been researched in the areas of:

    a) Alcohol misuse.
    b) Substance misuse.

c) Diet and exercise.
d) All of the above.

3. Motivational interviewing is a way of:

a) Tricking people into changing when they don't really want to.
b) Talking to people in an empathic and non-judgemental manner.
c) Getting people to see the error of their ways.
d) Coercing people to keep engaged with treatments that benefit them.

4. Motivational interviewing is a clinical method that:

a) Is based on the transtheoretical model of change.
b) Requires a set of standardised techniques.
c) Is a directive, empathic method for enhancing change by exploring and resolving ambivalence.
d) Requires a decisional balance sheet.

5. How might motivational interviewing need to be adapted to work with individuals who have complex and enduring mental health problems?

a) Simplification of open-ended questions.
b) Simplification of reflections and avoidance of reflection of disturbing content.
c) Increased amounts of affirmations to address issues of social stigma, lack of validation and frustration.
d) All of the above.

6. What are the key principles that underpin motivational interviewing?

a) Expressing empathy, developing discrepancy, rolling with resistance and supporting self-efficacy.
b) Expressing empathy, confronting client's behavioural choices, arguing for change and instructing people about what they ought to do.
c) Expressing empathy, instructing people about what they ought to do, rolling with resistance and supporting self-efficacy.
d) Instructing people about what they ought to do, confronting them with the error of their ways, coercing them into behaviour change and arguing with them about the need to change for their own benefit.

7. Ambivalence can be dealt with by:

a) Ignoring it because it might go away.
b) Directly confronting it by arguing that the client needs to make up her mind, one way or the other.
c) Empathising about how uncomfortable feeling ambivalent can be whilst also eliciting and exploring change talk.
d) Using decisional balance to weigh up the pros and cons of change.

8. The evidence base for using motivational interviewing methods to explore and resolve behaviour change for people with physical health problems and complex mental health needs:

a) Is as well developed as the evidence base for using motivational interviewing to address alcohol and substance misuse issues.
b) Does not look promising in assisting behaviour change in these areas.

*(Continued)*

*(Continued)*

    c) Has shown some promising results and should begin to be incorporated into treatment protocols to address these issues.

    d) Is too complex for either therapists or clients to attempt to use.

9. When resistance is encountered within a conversation about change, the best thing that a therapist can do is:

    a) Ignore it and hope it goes away.

    b) Argue with the client until you've convinced him to change his mind.

    c) Look for opportunities to respond by reflecting to the client about the resistance.

    d) See resistance as a sign that the therapy is not going to work and discharge the client as soon as possible.

10. When providing service users with information about health and healthy lifestyles, practitioners should:

    a) Insist that they read the information because they will be tested on it at their next appointment.

    b) Attempt to persuade them that the information they have given them is accurate and should not be disagreed with.

    c) Ask permission to provide information, ask what the service user already knows about the issue, provide information that is tailored to the service user's current knowledge, then ask about the service user's response to the information provided.

    d) Make sure that the information is provided in a glossy and attractive format.

# INTRODUCTION

Motivational interviewing is a client-centred, yet directive, method for enhancing intrinsic motivation to change by exploring and resolving service user ambivalence (Miller and Rollnick, 2002). Although initially focusing on the treatment of alcohol and substance misuse, in recent years motivational interviewing has been applied to address a wide range of clinical issues, including, among others, diet and exercise. Notwithstanding that a meta-analysis which included 132 empirical studies concluded that 117 (87%) of them targeted substance misuse, 15 of these studies (11%) focused primarily on helping people to increase healthy behaviours. There is no doubt that most of the evidence for the efficacy of motivational interviewing's efficacy is heavily weighted towards substance misuse and the efficacy for problem areas other than 'addictions' is sparse (Lundahl and Burke, 2009). However, motivational interviewing has begun to show particular promise in areas as diverse as HIV viral load, dental outcomes, death rate, body weight, alcohol and tobacco use, sedentary behaviour, self-monitoring, confidence in change and approach to treatment (Lundahl et al., 2013). There is still much speculation about how to successfully adapt motivational interviewing principles to meet the needs of specific populations (Miller et al., 2007; Burke, 2011). However, because motivational interviewing is firmly rooted in the relationship-building principles of a humanistic approach to therapy (Rogers, 1951) and therefore engages people in a compassionate, empathic and honest manner, it seems well-suited to address the kind of complex physical health issues that affect so many service users with enduring mental health problems.

This chapter will present a definition of motivational interviewing and give a brief history of its clinical and theoretical development. This chapter will also review the evidence base for its efficacy and effectiveness; describe some of the clinical skills required for its successful application; and attempt to generalise these skills towards working with people who have co-morbid mental health and physical health problems. It will be highlighted how engaging in some form of health behaviour change might improve their quality of life and enhance their physical health, wellbeing and life expectancy.

# WHAT IS MOTIVATIONAL INTERVIEWING?

Miller and Rollnick (2002) state that before learning about, and while practising motivational interviewing, it is vital to understand the overall spirit and underlying assumptions that fundamentally underpin the method. Motivational interviewing respects and honours an individual's autonomy to choose. Through a process of collaboration, the practitioner evokes the person's intrinsic motivation and resources for change. There must be an implicit belief that such motivation and resourcefulness lies within each individual and can be evoked but must not be imposed. Miller and Rollnick emphasise the need for practitioners to genuinely believe in the powerful potential for change residing in their service users and for practitioners to attempt to release that potential in order to facilitate and enhance the natural change processes already within the individual. In order to release this potential, they outline the following four broad guiding principles towards greater specificity of practice:

- Express empathy.
- Develop discrepancy.
- Roll with resistance.
- Support self-efficacy.

Each of these principles will be explored in more depth later in this chapter and their clinical applications discussed.

The intended focus of motivational interviewing is on those struggles where the individual is either not ready or willing for change or is displaying ambivalence about change. Being not ready or willing to consider change and, in particular, being ambivalent about whether to change or not, is a common enough experience for almost everyone to be able to relate to. Indeed, it is difficult to imagine a person who has never been ambivalent about something in their lives. We would guess that at least some of you reading this book might be feeling ambivalent right now about whether you want to read any more about motivational interviewing and whether motivational interviewing might prove to be useful as a method to be employed by you when, and if, you attempt to improve the physical health needs of the service users in your care.

Your ambivalence towards motivational interviewing might increase if we next tell you that motivational interviewing is not a simple set of techniques to be easily learnt and applied in order to 'deal' with the kind of 'annoying' motivational problems encountered by health care professionals when we attempt to improve the physical health of our service users. Motivational interviewing is a way of being with people that lies in an underlying spirit of understanding and experiencing human nature by attempting to understand why people often find change difficult, and by finding ways of talking to them that tap into and enhances their intrinsic motivation to change (ibid.).

## ⚙️ REFLECTION POINT 12.1

Think about the service that you work in/have worked in most recently:

- Were you aware of any attempts to collaboratively engage service users in conversations about potential health behaviour change?
- Were/are any of the members of your team trained in and/or practising motivational interviewing?

## A BRIEF HISTORY OF MOTIVATIONAL INTERVIEWING

In a seminal paper, Miller (1983) began to outline a different approach to talking to problem drinkers about their drinking. He stated that the traditional model of motivation in problem drinkers attributes almost all motivational properties to the personality of the drinker. A belief was prominent within treatment models for problem drinkers that the problematic drinker must progress downwards to a certain point of deterioration ('hitting rock bottom') before becoming somehow 'ready' for treatment. Over a period of eight years of working with problem drinkers, he developed what he describes as an 'intuitive' approach to talking to them about their alcohol issues. When students who observed his practice began to question why he behaved in radically different ways to the 'traditional' manner, he only then began to formalise his understanding of motivation and how to become more specific in his methods.

At first, because his novel approach lacked empirical evidence to support its efficacy, he was naturally tentative in his suggestions that it might be 'a' way to talk to 'some' individuals in a more useful manner. However, even in this early writing Miller was beginning to explore and develop the fundamental principles of the 'motivational interviewing approach'. Along with Rollnick and others, Miller began to incorporate recognised concepts from psychology, such as Festiner's (1957) theory of cognitive dissonance and Rogers' (1951, 1959, 1961) vitally important development of client-centred therapy. In other words, the clinical practice preceded the theories that ultimately underpin the approach and arose directly from Miller's own experience of talking to problem drinkers. The first full exposition of the method of motivational interviewing was published by Miller and Rollnick in 1991 and included the importance of 'working with ambivalence' as being at the heart of the motivational interviewing approach. It was here that motivational interviewing was first defined as: 'a client-centred, directive method for enhancing intrinsic motivation to change by exploring and resolving ambivalence' (ibid.: 22).

Since then, Miller, Rollnick and many other colleagues have developed, modified and refined the motivational interviewing approach into a living, breathing and ever-changing method for enhancing intrinsic motivation for change by exploring and helping to resolve ambivalence in their service users. In 2009, Miller and Rollnick attempted to address the confusion of motivational interviewing with Prochaska and DiClemente's very influential transtheoretical model of change (Prochaska and DiClemente, 1984; see below). At the same time, they addressed various other things that motivational interviewing is not (Miller and Rollnick, 2009). In 2015, Miller and Rose described two conceptually distinct methods for responding to ambivalence: decisional balance and the evocation of change talk. Although in the early descriptions of motivational interviewing, the use of decisional balance was propounded as an important element in this approach by giving equal attention to exploring both the 'pros' and 'cons' of both the status quo and change, they now cogently argue that, from a motivational interviewing perspective, if evoking a person's self-motivational reasons to change is the path out of ambivalence, then causing the individual to voice arguments against change would be contraindicated. They conclude, therefore, that using decisional balance is appropriate when practitioners wish to remain 'neutral' about whether the person should change or not. However, if practitioners wish to help service users resolve ambivalence in the direction of change, evocation is a much more useful method. Ambivalent service users, therefore, do not require the decisional balance approach, because it might make change less likely, whilst those individuals who are already planning to change might benefit from a decisional balance approach.

## THE TRANSTHEORETICAL MODEL OF CHANGE ('CYCLE OF CHANGE'; PROCHASKA AND DICLEMENTE, 1984)

Although, as previously mentioned, a clear distinction must be made between motivational interviewing and the transtheoretical model of change (or 'cycle of change', Prochaska and DiClemente, 1984), it is understandable that there remains confusion that the two things are one and the same (Miller and Rollnick, 2009). Both emerged together in the early 1980s.

The transtheoretical model, rather than being a manually driven therapy in its own right, offers a clinically useful framework for understanding key dimensions of behaviour change (DiClemente et al., 2011). The dimensions of change described by the transtheoretical model, including the different stages of change and common components of change for individuals within these different stages, offer a structure for understanding how and why individuals may or may not change.

The stages of change can be summarised as follows: pre-contemplation, contemplation, preparation, action, maintenance, relapse.

## PRE-CONTEMPLATION

Pre-contemplators can be summarised as not at present seeing the need for lifestyle or behaviour change. They often present in several different ways. Reluctant, rebellious, resigned or rationalising pre-contemplators are all commonly seen, and all must be addressed with empathy, whilst attempting to raise interest, concern and increased awareness of the current situation.

## CONTEMPLATION

Contemplators are beginning to consider that change might be a possibility but might be some way from any kind of commitment to change. The tasks for practitioners might include helping to weigh the 'pros and cons' of change. However, caution should be taken whilst doing this, because an unfortunate consequence of weighing up evidence for and against change might be to reinforce the status quo (Miller and Rose, 2015).

## PREPARATION

Individuals who are preparing to change, having begun to make up their mind to attempt to change, require assistance to develop realistic, achievable and potentially effective plans for change.

## ACTION

At this stage, individuals can be assisted with implementing agreed plans and require help to address potential barriers of all kinds.

## MAINTENANCE

Individuals now need to find ways to incorporate behaviour change into their everyday lives, whilst finding ways to address the possibility of relapse into previous patterns of behaviour.

## RELAPSE

An important component of the transtheoretical model is an explicit acknowledgement that relapse, although, of course, not inevitable, is usual and not unexpected. It is seen as an opportunity to review plans and preparations for change. The practitioner can destigmatise relapse by stressing its ubiquity and by using it as an opportunity to enhance future change plans.

---

### ⚙ REFLECTION POINT 12.2

- In regard to your own physical wellbeing, where would you place yourself on the 'cycle of change' if you were to consider addressing your own relationship to diet and exercise?
- Think about several different service users on your current caseload. Could you, with the information about them that you already have, make a reasonably accurate guess about where they would be on the 'cycle of change' if you were to have a conversation with them about improving their lifestyles to incorporate a more healthy approach to diet and exercise?
- Where would you place your own service if you were to attempt to define it in the 'cycle of change'?

---

# THE EVIDENCE BASE FOR MOTIVATIONAL INTERVIEWING

Since its inception as a way of talking to people about behaviour change, there has been a large and constantly growing evidence base for motivational interviewing. Attempts have been made to explore in a systematic manner why and how people might change (Apodaca and Longabaugh, 2009); and the relevant principles from social psychology have been reviewed (Leffingwell et al., 2007). The efficacy for utilising motivational interviewing when treating alcohol and substance use disorders has been clearly demonstrated (Lundahl and Burke, 2009). More recently, motivational interviewing and related interventions have been researched to see whether they can be applied to a variety of other clinical problems, including the treatment of psychological problems (Arkowitz et al., 2008), and the treatment of a wide variety of conditions in medical care settings, including dental outcomes, body weight, alcohol and tobacco use and sedentary behaviour (Lundahl et al., 2013). Additionally, a number of studies have been undertaken to explore the efficacy of motivational interviewing with a range of client groups in a variety of different clinical settings: substance use within psychiatric inpatient services (Baker et al., 2002); alcohol use with depressed and anxious people; cannabis use among people with serious mental disorders (ibid., 2009); 'dually diagnosed' individuals

(Barrowclough et al., 2010; Martino et al., 2006); schizophrenia and alcohol misuse (Graeber et al., 2003); and substance misuse in recent onset of psychosis (Kavanagh et al., 2004).

In brief, motivational interviewing is now seen as an efficacious and effective treatment modality to help people to address health behaviour change in a way that is empathic, honest, non-judgemental and person-centred. There has also been a concerted effort to systematically review the efficacy of training health professionals in the delivery of motivational interviewing approaches (Barwick et al., 2012; Decker and Martino, 2013; de Roten et al., 2013), which will be discussed later in this chapter.

# THE CLINICAL APPLICATION OF MOTIVATIONAL INTERVIEWING

This chapter is not able to discuss in depth or detail the complex and multifaceted components of motivational interviewing or give huge amounts of detail about how and when to apply it. However, the tasks involved in its clinical application have been summarised as follows (Miller and Moyers, 2006):

- Understanding and using the 'spirit' of motivational interviewing.
- Using client-centred skills (OARS; see below).
- Recognising change talk.
- Eliciting and reinforcing change talk.
- Rolling with resistance.
- Developing a change plan.
- Consolidating service user commitment to change.
- Integrating motivational interviewing with other intervention methods.

---

### 👤👤👤   CASE STUDY 12.1

Dennis is 31 years old. Ten years ago, he experienced a first episode of a psychotic illness while in full-time education. He was doing an access course at a local further education college when his illness began. He withdrew from his course immediately and there has been no further contact with the college.

He initially presented with a range of 'positive' symptoms of psychosis – hearing derogatory and commanding voices, experiencing distressing persecutory beliefs and having trouble ordering his thoughts. Since this initial episode, his 'positive' psychotic symptoms have responded well to treatment. However, although he remains on regular oral medication, olanzapine 20 mg daily, he has become increasingly withdrawn. He seldom leaves his house and his old group of friends seldom visit as he never contacts them.

Prior to the first onset of his psychotic illness, Dennis used to have all kinds of interests and abilities. He used to play for a Sunday League football team and trained with them once a week. He also liked to use the gym at his old college because he prided himself on his fitness. However, he now finds that the local gym is too intimidating an environment for him to handle and he has stopped doing any exercises at home. He has put on over 25 kg within months of commencing olanzapine and now leads an increasingly sedentary lifestyle. His only current activity is watching TV alone at home. His lack of activity causes arguments between Dennis and his mum, because she believes that he could be doing much more with his time. However, when questioned about what he wants to do, he finds it hard to come up with any new ideas. He is pessimistic about the future and doesn't think he'll ever be able to initiate changes in his current lifestyle.

Dennis was referred by his care coordinator for motivational interviewing to address his ambivalence about change. The initial meeting established several important and useful considerations. When the practitioner discussed the *importance* of changing his current sedentary lifestyle, Dennis rated this as 8/10, because he was aware of the physical health risks associated with his current lifestyle and could remember a time when he had enjoyed being physically active. His stated *goal* was to be able to increase his activity and to lose weight. However, his *confidence* about being able to change was rated as 2/10.

Over two subsequent sessions, the practitioner explored Dennis's current ambivalence about change by employing a motivational conversational style. Reflections were used to explore his ambivalence about change and to highlight the dichotomy between Dennis's stated goals and his current behaviour. He was asked how much his confidence would have to increase before he was willing to begin to initiate a health behaviour change. He stated that it would need to increase to at least 6/10. By the end of two sessions of motivational interviewing, his confidence appeared to have increased, mainly by the promotion of self-efficacy and by enabling him to remember a time when he was fit and active, including how much he used to enjoy regular exercise. This enabled his care team to plan and deliver an individualised exercise programme (see Chapter 7 for how to develop such a programme) in order to enable Dennis to re-establish activities that he had previously engaged in and enjoyed.

## THE SPIRIT OF MOTIVATIONAL INTERVIEWING

An essential component of motivational interviewing is the spirit that underpins it. It can be simplified into the following categories: autonomy, collaboration and evocation.

### AUTONOMY

- Honour expertise, which resides within the individual. Be mindful of both parties' positions. It is not authoritarian.
- Talk less than them.
- Help them to straighten things out for themselves.

## COLLABORATION

- Resource for motivation and change lies with the individual, the practitioner affirms and supports this.
- It is not confrontational.
- Invite them to talk.

## EVOCATION

- Motivation for change is enhanced by elicitation, rather than persuasion or instilling.
- Listen to their answers and listen out for talk about change.
- Encourage them on their way.

# PRINCIPLES OF MOTIVATIONAL INTERVIEWING

## EXPRESS EMPATHY

- Ambivalence is normal.
- Expressing empathy for this ambivalence is vital.

## SUPPORT SELF-EFFICACY

- The service user is responsible for change and must believe that it is possible.
- People whose workers believe that they are likely to change do so. Those who are told that they are expected to change don't.

## ROLL WITH RESISTANCE

- Avoid arguments.
- View resistance as a sign to respond differently.
- Respond with reflection and empathic listening.

## DEVELOP DISCREPANCY

- Support the service user to review arguments for change in relation to their core values.
- Empathic conversations will elicit the individual's goals and values and help them to consider these goals in relation to their current behaviour.

In addition to the spirit that underpins motivational interviewing and the principles that guide this method for talking to people about health behaviour change, the intervention requires the strategic use of essential skills. The essential skills in motivational interviewing are often referred to as OARS (see Table 12.1).

**Table 12.1   Open Affirm Reflect Summarise (OARS)**

| | |
|---|---|
| O | Use **OPEN** questions to explore the possibility of changing |
| A | **AFFIRM** what the service user is saying is important |
| R | **REFLECT** what the service user is saying. Reflections can be simple or complex. One of the key skills in motivational interviewing is not only being able to reflect, but in being able to choose, where possible, the right type of reflection at the right time. Different types of reflection include: repeating, rephrasing, paraphrasing, double-sided reflections, agreement with a twist, shifting focus and amplified reflection. All have a purpose if used in the right place at the right time. This purpose is to attempt to resolve ambivalence and to begin to elicit and enhance change talk |
| S | **SUMMARISE** what the service user is saying. This makes sure they know they've been truly heard, whilst ensuring that you've heard exactly what you think you have |

## AMBIVALENCE

Ambivalence is normal when considering change (Miller and Rose, 2015). It is characteristic of the 'contemplation' stage of change. People often experience motivations both for and against change, often simultaneously. The following statements are typical of ambivalence:

- I need to lose some weight but I hate doing exercise.
- I should quit smoking but I just can't seem to be able to do so.
- At the end of our sessions, I always mean to do what we've suggested but when it comes down to it, I just forget to do it.

The following questions are either explicit or implicit when people are ambivalent:

- Should I change? (Importance)
- Can I change? (Confidence, self-efficacy)
- Will I fail? (Lack of confidence)
- Will I fail again? (Lack of confidence based on previous experiences of failure)

The best way to respond to ambivalence is by using OARS.

## CHANGE TALK

People who are beginning to resolve ambivalence in the direction of positive change will begin to express questions such as:

- Will I change? (Commitment)
- How do I go about changing? (Options, strategies)
- How do I maintain changes I've made? (Continuing commitment)

The strategic emphasis in motivational interviewing is on attempting to elicit change talk, in other words those self-generated arguments by the service user on behalf of change, and to strengthen them if possible; and by responding to sustain talk (the reasons for not changing) by showing respect for them but avoiding strengthening them. The different ways that people might express change talk have been simplified to 'DARN-C' (Table 12.2).

**Table 12.2   Desire Ability Reasons Need-Commitments (DARN-C)**

| | |
|---|---|
| D | **Desire:** Statements that show a preference towards change ('I really want to begin to make some changes to my diet') |
| A | **Ability:** Statements that display increased confidence in the capability to change ('I know I can do it next time; I've already decided what diet I'm going to try and it doesn't look too hard') |
| R | **Reasons:** Specific arguments for change ('I want to be able to play with my grandchildren without getting out of breath and being a bit fitter would really help') |
| N | **Need:** Statements expressing an obligation to change, often externally generated ('My girlfriend says she'll leave me if I don't lose some weight and start to improve my appearance') |
| C | **Commitment:** 'I will change; this time, I'm going to do it and to stick with it' |

We need to respond to change talk in specific ways, all of which aim to reinforce it and to strengthen it. Elaboration ('tell me more'); affirmation ('that sounds like an excellent plan'); reflection ('you seem to have really thought this through'); and summaries ('so you've decided to change your eating habits, you've chosen your diet, you've researched how you'll buy and cook your new diet and you've thought about some potential obstacles which might stop you. It looks like you've got every chance now').

## *RESISTANCE*

Resistance is inevitable. It arises, to a significant degree, from the interpersonal inter-action between practitioner and service user (Miller and Rollnick, 2002). It represents an important sign of dissonance within the therapeutic process. It shows that the service user no longer agrees with you or is maybe not even on the same page as you, with a different world view, a different agenda from you or a different idea of how to behave from you. How a practitioner responds to resistance is a key feature of motivational interviewing. Practitioners can respond to resistance in ways that either increase it or decrease. Obviously, the imperative is to attempt to respond to it in ways that decrease it if possible or at least to acknowledge its existence.

As Miller and Rollnick state: 'A good general principle is to respond to resist-ance with non-resistance' (2002: 100). The acknowledgement of an individual's disagreement permits further and alternative explanation rather than continued defensiveness by the practitioner, to avoid the trap of taking sides. Simple reflections will often be appropriate, including reflection of feelings, for example: 'You sound like you're fed up and angry about what I've just said.' However, often more complex reflections can be very helpful to avoid further resistance. For instance, an amplified reflection can be very useful – reflecting back a resistant remark in an amplified or exaggerated form. This may encourage the individual to back off from resistance and instead allow them to respond to the amplification by eliciting a response expressing the other side of ambivalence, for example: 'I couldn't imagine being able to change my diet. All my friends mainly eat takeaways, too.' 'So you couldn't handle what your mates would say if you didn't go with them to the takeaway?' Other, more complex, forms of reflection include double-sided reflections, for example: 'So, on the one hand, you think that increasing exercise might really help you to lose weight, but on the other hand it's hard to imagine getting started.' Shifting focus, reframing and agreeing with a twist are also useful ways of responding to resistance and they all avoid argumentation. Miller and Rollnick (ibid.) discuss the 'drama' of change, with resistance becoming a key to successful treatment if it is seen as an opportunity to 'change the usual script' that a service user has rehearsed so many times before. By responding in unexpected and reflective ways to resistance, the plot gets potentially changed and new conversations about the possibility of change may emerge.

---

### ⚙ REFLECTION POINT 12.3

Reflect for a few minutes on service users whom you have worked with who appear to be making poor choices about their lifestyles or who show signs of struggling to care for their own physical health. Do you think that these service users should be encouraged to improve their physical health? If they resist your attempts to offer them the opportunity to engage in healthy lifestyle changes, how would you feel? How would you respond to signs of resistance to change?

---

## PROVISION OF INFORMATION

Motivational interviewing principles and the spirit that underpins them present some genuinely useful ways of providing information to people about physical ill health and ways to improve it. Providing information on a range of health issues is, of course, a very important part of any health professional's role and responsibility. Done badly, it will provide information that is possibly not relevant, pitched at a level or in a format that is not accessible or acceptable to the service user and potentially contradicts their own existing attitudes, values and knowledge. Hence, this information provision may leave the service user feeling patronised, ignored, contradicted or humiliated by a so-called 'expert'. This, in turn, is likely to lead to resistance, both to the information provided and to future attempts at empathy and collaborative engagement. However, if done well, it will result in better understanding and enhanced therapeutic alliance (Rollnick et al., 1999).

Information provision can be greatly improved by using the 'Permission – Ask – Provide – Ask' method or PAPA (Hettema and Kirsch, 2011; see Table 12.3).

### Table 12.3    Permission Ask Provide Ask (PAPA)

| | |
|---|---|
| P | **Permission:** 'I'd like to give you some information about the benefits of increased exercise; is that OK with you?' |
| A | **Ask:** 'What do you already know about the benefits of increased exercise? Have you got any previous experience of increasing exercise? Do you know anyone who has attempted to do more exercise?' |
| P | **Provide:** 'You've told me that you tend not to like to read written material; so, here's a short DVD about the benefits of increased exercise. It would be good if you could find time to watch it before we meet again next week. Is there anything that's likely to prevent you from doing so?' |
| A | **Ask:** 'How did you find the DVD? Was there anything that you found useful? Was there anything you disagreed with? Is there now anything else you'd like to know?' |

## CAN MOTIVATIONAL INTERVIEWING BE EFFECTIVE IN ENHANCING HEALTH BEHAVIOUR CHANGE?

As anyone reading this book will already be only too aware, the physical health needs of people with mental health problems is a hugely important issue that is only now beginning to be addressed. It is therefore vital that anyone working towards improving physical health in this client group must be able to find effective evidence-based ways of discussing these issues that enhance the chances of change occurring. These conversations often occur when the practitioner usually wants to talk about health behaviour change with a service user who might appear to lack motivation to change (Rollnick et al., 1999).

As previously stated, most of the evidence to support the efficacy of motivational interviewing has been undertaken to address issues of alcohol and other psychoactive substance misuse, including heroin, cocaine and cannabis. However, there has also been some promising research into its application to enhance health behaviour change to address other issues, such as smoking cessation and the promotion of healthier lifestyles, including dietary improvement and increase in exercise. Lundahl et al. (2010) summarise some of these studies in a systematic review and meta-analysis. They report promising results in areas such as dental outcomes, body weight, tobacco use and sedentary behaviour. However, few studies have so far featured service users who have complex mental health problems. One example was undertaken by Steinberg et al. (2004). These authors trialled a brief intervention using motivational interviewing to improve motivation in smokers with schizophrenia to engage in treatment for tobacco dependence. A more recent feasibility study to introduce a counselling and exercise intervention for service users with a diagnosis of schizophrenia, which employed a single group prospective design, reported promising findings regarding smoking reduction and appeared to be both feasible and acceptable to participants (Bernard et al., 2013). Unfortunately, the lack of a control group makes it difficult to draw any firm conclusions about the efficacy of this intervention.

Despite the dearth of evidence in this field, it is worth remaining optimistic about the use of motivational interviewing to address issues of health behaviour change in service users with mental health problems. It has already featured in promising trials for people with a 'dual diagnosis' of co-existing substance misuse and mental ill health (Drake et al., 2007).

## CONCLUSION

Health professionals often find themselves talking to their service users about potential health behaviour change. These professionals sometimes find this a disempowering and demoralising activity, where changes are often perceived as glacially slow or non-existent. These professionals normally have their service users' best interest at heart and try to carry out their health promotion roles with diligence and determination. In their frustration, the temptation is often to attempt persuasion, coercion or even frightening people, in the hope that this will result in the desired change. However, by employing the core principles of motivational interviewing, including expressing empathy about ambivalence and acknowledging that change is difficult, supporting the service user's self-efficacy, rolling with resistance and developing discrepancy, and underpinning those principles by remaining congruent to the spirit of motivational interviewing through collaboration, support for autonomy and evocation, there is the potential to enhance health behaviour change whilst fostering open and honest relationships with service users.

## USEFUL RESOURCES

Matulich, B. (2013) *Introduction to Motivational Interviewing*. Available at: www.youtube.com/watch?v=s3MCJZ7OGRk (accessed 3 October 2016 ).

This brief YouTube video provides a balanced summary introduction to motivational interviewing.

Motivational Interviewing Network of Trainers (MINT) website. Available at: www.motivationalinterviewing.org.

This is an accessible and highly informative website that links the reader to resources and training opportunities on offer from MINT. The exercises available for training purposes are wide-ranging and accessible for use by individuals and groups.

## ANSWERS TO MULTIPLE CHOICE QUESTIONS

1(d), 2(d), 3(b), 4(c), 5(d), 6(a), 7(c), 8(c), 9(c), 10(c)

# REFERENCES

Action on Smoking and Health (ASH) (2016) *The Stolen Years: The Mental Health and Smoking Action Report*. Available at: www.ash.org.uk/current-policy-issues/health-inequalities/smoking-and-mental-health/the-stolen-years (accessed 25 August 2016).

Adams, D.J., Remick, R.A., Davis, J.C. et al. (2015) 'Exercise as medicine – the use of group medical visits to promote physical activity and treat chronic moderate depression: a preliminary 14-week pre-post study', *BMJ Open Sport and Exercise Medicine*, 1: e000036. Available at: http://bmjopensem.bmj.com/content/1/1/e000036.full.pdf+html (accessed 25 August 2016).

Addington, J. and Haarmans, M. (2006) 'Cognitive-Behavioral Therapy for individuals recovering from a first episode of psychosis', *Journal of Contemporary Psychotherapy*, 36 (1): 43–49.

Addington, J., Saeedi, H. and Addington, D. (2006) 'Weight gain in first-episode psychosis over three years', *Schizophrenia Research*, 86: 335–6.

Addington, J., Case, N., Saleem, M.M. et al. (2014) 'Substance use in clinical high risk for psychosis: a review of the literature', *Early Intervention in Psychiatry*, 8(2): 104–12.

Addington, J., Cornblatt, B.A., Cadenhead, K.S. et al. (2011) 'At clinical high risk for psychosis: outcome for nonconverters', *American Journal of Psychiatry*, 168(8): 80–5.

Alberti, K., Zimmet, P., Shaw, J. and Epidemiology Task Force Consensus Group (2005) 'The metabolic syndrome: a new worldwide definition', *The Lancet*, 366: 1059–62.

Alfonsson, S., Parling, T. and Ghaderi, A. (2015) 'Group behavioral activation for patients with severe obesity and binge eating disorder: a randomized controlled trial', *Behavior Modification*, 39(2): 270–94.

Álvarez-Jiménez, M., Gleeson, J., Henry, L. et al. (2012) 'Road to full recovery: longitudinal relationship between symptomatic remission and psychosocial recovery in first-episode psychosis over 7.5 years', *Psychological Medicine*, 42: 595–606.

Álvarez-Jiménez, M., Gonzalez-Blanch, C., Crespo-Facorro, B. et al. (2008) 'Antipsychotic-induced weight gain in chronic and first episode psychotic disorders: a systematic critical reappraisal', *CNS Drugs*, 22: 547–62.

Amminger, G.P., Schäfer, M.R., Papageorgiou, K. et al. (2010) 'Long-chain omega-3 fatty acids for indicated prevention of psychotic disorders: a randomized, placebo-controlled trial', *Arch. Gen. Psychiatry*, 67(2): 146–54.

Amminger, G.P., Schäfer, M.R., Schlögelhofer, M. et al. (2015) 'Longer-term outcome in the prevention of psychotic disorders by the Vienna omega-3 study', *Nature Communications*, 6. http://dx.doi.org/10.1038/ncomms8934 (accessed 25 August 2016).

Andrews, P.W., Anderson Thomson, J., Amstadter, A. and Neale, M.C. (2012) '*Primum non nocere*: an evolutionary analysis of whether antidepressants do more harm than good', *Frontiers in Psychology*, 3(117): 1–19.

Apodaca, T.R. and Longabaugh, R. (2009) 'Mechanisms of change in MI: a review and preliminary evaluation of the evidence', *Addiction*, 104: 705–15.

Appleby, L. (2008) Conference address to Policies and Practices for Mental Health in Europe: Meeting the Challenges, Department of Health and World Health Organization Europe Conference attended by 35 countries, 10 October, London.

Arango, C., Garibaldi, G. and Marder, S.R. (2013) 'Pharmacological approaches to treating negative symptoms: a review of clinical trials', *Schizophrenia Research*, 150: 346–52.

Archie, S., Wilson, J.H., Osborne, S. et al. (2003) 'Pilot study: access to fitness facility and levels in olanzapine-treated patients', *Can. J. Psychiatry/La Revue canadienne de psychiatrie*, 48: 628–32.

Arkowitz, H., Westra, H.A., Miller, W.R. and Rollnick, S. (2008) *Motivational Interviewing in the Treatment of Psychological Problems*. New York: Guilford Press.

Auther, A., McLaughlin, D., Carrion, R. et al. (2012) 'Prospective study of cannabis use in adolescents at clinical high risk for psychosis: impact on conversion to psychosis and functional outcome', *Psychological Medicine*, 42(12): 2485–97.

Aveyard, P., Begh, R., Parsons, A. and West, R. (2012) 'Brief opportunistic smoking cessation interventions: a systematic review and meta-analysis to compare advice to quit and offer of assistance', *Addiction*, 107: 1066–73.

Bailey, S., Gerada, C., Lester, H. and Shiers, D. (2012) 'The cardiovascular health of young people with severe mental illness: addressing an epidemic within an epidemic', *The Psychiatrist*, 36: 375–8.

Baker, A., Turner, A., Kay-Lambkin, F.J. and Lewin, T.J. (2009) 'The long and the short of treatments for alcohol or cannabis misuse among people with severe mental disorders', *Addictive Behaviours*, 34: 852–8.

Baker, A., Lewin, T., Reichler, H. et al. (2002) 'Evaluation of motivational interview for substance use within psychiatric inpatient services', *Journal of Addiction*, 97(10): 1329–37.

Banham, L. and Gilbody, S.M. (2010) 'Smoking cessation in severe mental illness: what works?', *Addiction*, 105: 1176–89.

Bänziger, S., Hegedü, S.A., Burr, C. et al. (2016) 'Einsatz des Gesundheitsförderungsprofils Psychiatrie GEPPSY zur Erhebung körperlicher Gesundheitsrisiken von Menschen mit schweren psychischen Erkrankungen im ambulanten Setting', *Pflegewissenschaft*, 18: 125–33.

Barber, J., Palmese, L., Reutenauer, E.L. et al. (2011) 'Implications of weight-based stigma and self-bias on quality of life among individuals with schizophrenia', *Journal of Nervous and Mental Disease*, 199: 431–5.

Barnes, T.R. and the Schizophrenia Consensus Group of British Association for Psychopharmacology (2011) 'Evidence-based guidelines for the pharmacological treatment of schizophrenia: recommendations from the British Association for Psychopharmacology', *Journal of Psychopharmacology*, 25: 567–620.

Barnett, A., Mackin, P., Chaudhry, I. et al. (2007) 'Minimizing metabolic and cardiovascular risk in schizophrenia: diabetes, obesity and dyslipidaemia', *Journal of Psychopharmacology*, 21: 357–73.

Barrowclough, C., Haddock, G., Wykes T. et al. (2010) 'Integrated motivational interviewing and cognitive behavioural therapy for people with psychosis and co-morbid substance misuse: randomised controlled trial', *BMJ*. Available at: www.bmj.com/content/bmj/341/bmj.c6325.full.pdf (accessed 25 August 2016).

Bartels, S.J. (2015) 'Can behavioral health organizations change health behaviors? The STRIDE study and lifestyle interventions for obesity in serious mental illness', *American Journal of Psychiatry*, 172: 9–11.

Bartels, S.J., Pratt, S.I., Aschbrenner, K.A. et al. (2013) 'Clinically significant improved fitness and weight loss among overweight persons with serious mental illness', *Psychiatric Services*, 64: 729–36.

Barwick, M.A., Bennett, L.M., Johnson, S.N. et al. (2012) 'Training health and mental health professionals in motivational interviewing: a systematic review', *Children and Youth Services Review*, 34: 1786–95.

Bass, C., and Mayou, R. (2002) 'Chest pain', *BMJ*, 325: 588–91.

Bernard, P.P.N., Esseul, E.C., Raymond, L. et al. (2013) 'Counseling and exercise intervention for smoking reduction in patients with schizophrenia: a feasibility study', *Archives of Psychiatric Nursing*, 27: 23–31.

Bhaskaran, K., Douglas, I., Forbes, H. et al. (2014) 'Body mass index and risk of 22 specific cancers: a population-based cohort study of 5.24 million UK adults', *The Lancet*, 384(9945): 755–65.

Black, M.H., Sacks, D.A., Xiang, A.H. and Lawrence, J.M. (2013) 'The relative contribution of prepregnancy overweight and obesity, gestational weight gain, and IADPSG-defined gestational diabetes mellitus to fetal overgrowth', *Diabetes Care*, 36(1): 56–62.

Blair, S.N. (2009) 'Physical inactivity: the biggest public health problem of the 21st century', *British Journal of Sports Medicine*, 43: 1–2.

Blumenthal, S.R., Castro, V.M., Clements, C.M.S. et al. (2014) 'An electronic health records study of long-term weight gain following antidepressant use', *JAMA Psychiatry*, 71(8): 889–96.

Bonfioli, E.L., Berti, L., Goss, C. et al. (2012) 'Health promotion lifestyle interventions for weight management in psychosis: a systematic review and meta-analysis of randomised controlled trials', *BMC Psychiatry*, 12: 78.

Bordin, E.S. (1979) 'The generalisability of the psychoanalytic concept of the working alliance', *Psychotherapy: Theory, Research and Practice*, 16(3): 252.

Bowers, K., Laughon, S.K., Kiely, M. et al. (2013) 'Gestational diabetes, pre-pregnancy obesity and pregnancy weight gain in relation to excess fetal growth: variations by race/ethnicity', *Diabetologia*, 56: 1263–71.

Bowie, C.R., Grossman, M., Gupta, M. et al. (2014) 'Cognitive remediation in schizophrenia: efficacy and effectiveness in patients with early versus long-term course of illness', *Early Intervention in Psychiatry*, 8: 32–8.

Bradshaw, T. and Mairs, H. (2014) 'Obesity and serious mental ill health: a critical review of the literature', *Healthcare*, Special Edition, *The Burden of Obesity in Health Care*, 2: 166–82.

Bradshaw, T., Wearden, A., Marshall, M. et al. (2012) 'Developing a healthy living intervention for people with early psychosis using the Medical Research Council's guidelines on complex interventions: Phase 1 of the HELPER – InterACT programme', *International Journal of Nursing Studies*, 49: 398–406.

Bressington, D.T., Mui, J., Cheung, E.F. et al. (2013) 'The prevalence of metabolic syndrome amongst patients with severe mental illness in the community in Hong Kong: a cross-sectional study', *BMC Psychiatry*, 13: 87.

Bressington, D., Mui, J., Hulbert, S. et al. (2014) 'Enhanced physical health screening for people with severe mental illness in Hong Kong: results from a one-year prospective case series study', *BMC Psychiatry*, 14: 57.

Bressington, D., Mui, J., Wells, H. et al. (2016) 'Refocusing on physical health: community psychiatric nurses' perceptions of using enhanced health checks for people with severe mental illness', *Int. J. Ment. Health Nurs*. Available at: www.ncbi.nlm.nih.gov/pubmed/26857108 (accessed 25 August 2016).

Briscoe, V.J. and Davis, S.N. (2006) 'Hypoglycemia in type 1 and type 2 diabetes: physiology, pathophysiology, and management', *Clinical Diabetes*, 24: 115–21.

Brown, S., Kim, M., Mitchell, C. and Inskip, H. (2010) 'Twenty-five year mortality of a community cohort with schizophrenia', *British Journal of Psychiatry*, 196: 116–21.

Browne, J., Mihas, P. and Penn, D.L. (2015) 'Focus on exercise: client and clinician perspectives on exercise in individuals with serious mental illness', *Community Mental Health Journal*, 1–8: doi: 10.1007/s10597-015-9896-y.

Bruins, J., Jörg, F., Bruggeman, R. et al. (2014) 'The effects of lifestyle interventions on (long-term) weight management, cardiometabolic risk and depressive symptoms in people with psychotic disorders: a meta-analysis', *PLOS ONE*, 9(12): e112276. Doi: 10.1371/journal.pone.0112276.

Burke, B.L. (2011) 'What can Motivational Interviewing do for you?', *Cognitive and Behavioural Practice*, 18: 74–81.

Caemmerer, J., Correll, C.U. and Maayan, L. (2012) 'Acute and maintenance effects of non-pharmacologic interventions for antipsychotic associated weight gain and metabolic abnormalities: a meta-analytic comparison of randomized controlled trials', *Schizophr. Res.*, 140: 159–68.

Callaghan, R.C., Boire, M.D., Lazo, R.G. et al. (2009) 'Schizophrenia and the incidence of cardiovascular morbidity: a population-based longitudinal study in Ontario', *Canada Schizophrenia Research*, 115(2–3): 325–32.

Callaghan, R., Velhuizen, S., Jeysingh, T. et al. (2014) 'Patterns of tobacco-related mortality among individuals diagnosed with schizophrenia, bipolar disorder, or depression', *Journal of Psychiatric Research*, 48(1): 102–10.

Campion, J., Shiers, D., Britton, J. et al. (2014) *National Primary Care Guidance on Smoking and Mental Disorder*, 2014 update. Royal College of General Practitioners. Available at: http://rcpsych.ac.uk/pdf/PrimaryCareGuidanceonSmokingandMentalDisorders2014update.pdf (accessed 25 August 2016).

Carleton, R.N., Duranceau, S., Freeston, M.H. et al. (2014) '"But it might be a heart attack": intolerance of uncertainty and panic disorder symptoms', *Journal of Anxiety Disorders*, 28(5): 463–70.

Carney, R., Bradshaw, T. and Yung, A.R. (2015) 'Monitoring of physical health in services for young people at ultra-high risk of psychosis', *Early Intervention in Psychiatry*. Available at: http://onlinelibrary.wiley.com/doi/10.1111/eip.12288/epdf (accessed 25 August 2016).

Carney, R., Cotter, J., Bradshaw, T. et al. (2016) 'Cardiometabolic risk factors in young people at ultra-high risk for psychosis: a systematic review and meta-analysis', *Schizophrenia Research*, 170(2): 290–300.

Caspersen, C.J., Powell, K.E. and Christenson, G.M. (1985) 'Physical activity, exercise, and physical fitness: definitions and distinctions for health-related research', *Public Health Reports*, 100: 126.

Chastin, S.F., Palarea-Albaladejo, J., Dontje, M.L. and Skelton, D.A. (2015) 'Combined effects of time spent in physical activity, sedentary behaviors and sleep on obesity and cardio-metabolic health markers: a novel compositional data analysis approach', *PLOS ONE*, 10: e0139984.

Chesney, E., Goodwin, G.M. and Fazel, S. (2014) 'Risks of all-cause and suicide mortality in mental disorders: a meta-review', *World Psychiatry*. 13: 153–60.

Church, T.S., Blair, S.N., Cocreham, S. et al. (2010) 'Effects of aerobic and resistance training on hemoglobin A1c levels in patients with type 2 diabetes: a randomized controlled trial', *Jama*, 304: 2253–62.

Clancy, J. and McVicar, A.J. (2009) *Physiology and Anatomy for Nurses and Healthcare Practitioners*, 3rd edn. London: Hodder Arnold.

Commission on Chronic Illness (1957) *Chronic Illness in the United States*, Vol. 1: *Prevention of Chronic Illness*. London: Oxford University Press.

Connolly, M., Floyd, S., Forrest, R. and Marshall, B. (2013) 'Mental health nurses' beliefs about smoking by mental health facility inpatients', *International Journal of Mental Health Nursing*, 22: 288–93.

Cooney, G.M., Dwan, K., Greig, C.A. et al. (2013) 'Exercise for depression', *Cochrane Database Syst. Rev.* 9(9). Available at: http://onlinelibrary.wiley.com/doi/10.1002/14651858. CD004366.pub6/full (accessed 25 August 2016).

Correll, C.U., Robinson, D.G., Schooler, N.R. et al. (2014) 'Cardiometabolic risk in patients with first-episode schizophrenia spectrum disorders: Baseline results from the RAISE-ETP study', *JAMA Psychiatry*, 71: 1350–63.

Cotter, J., Drake, R.J., Bucci, S. et al. (2014) 'What drives poor functioning in the at-risk mental state? A systematic review', *Schizophrenia Research*, 159(2): 267–77.

Crawford, M.J., Jayakumar, S., Lemmey, S.J. et al. (2014) 'Assessment and treatment of physical health problems among people with schizophrenia: national cross-sectional study', *British Journal of Psychiatry*, 205: 473–7.

Cretikos, M.A., Bellomo, R., Hillman, K. et al. (2008) 'Respiratory rate: the neglected vital sign', *Medical Journal of Australia*, 188(11): 657–9.

Curtis, J., Newall, H. and Samaras, K. (2012) 'The heart of the matter: cardiometabolic care in youth with psychosis', *Early Intervention in Psychiatry*, 6: 347–53.

Curtis, J., Watkins, A. and Rosenbaum, S. (2014) 'Early lifestyle intervention attenuates antipsychotic-induced weight gain in first episode psychosis', *Early Intervention in Psychiatry*, 8: 30.

Curtis, J., Watkins, A., Rosenbaum, S. et al. (2015) 'Evaluating an individualized lifestyle and life skills intervention to prevent antipsychotic-induced weight gain in first-episode psychosis', *Early Intervention in Psychiatry*, published online 26 February: doi: 10.1111/eip.12230.

Daumit, G.L., Pratt, L.A., Crum, R.M. et al. (2002) 'Characteristics of primary care visits for individuals with severe mental illness in a national sample', *Gen. Hosp. Psychiatry*, 24: 391–5.

de Boer, M.K., Castelein, S., Wiersma, D. et al. (2014) 'The facts about sexual (dys)function in schizophrenia: an overview of clinically relevant findings – antipsychotic treatment and sexual functioning', *Schizophrenia Bulletin*, 41(3): 674–86.

De Hert, M., Detraux, J., van Winkel, R. et al. (2012) 'Metabolic and cardiovascular adverse effects associated with antipsychotic drugs', *Nature Reviews Endocrinology*, 8: 114–26.

De Hert, M.A., van Winkel, R., Van Eyck, D. et al. (2006) 'Prevalence of the metabolic syndrome in patients with schizophrenia treated with antipsychotic medication', *Schizophrenia Research*, 83: 87–93.

de Roten, Y., Zimmerman, G., Ortega, D. and Despland, J.N. (2013) 'Meta-analysis of the effects of MI training on clinicians' behaviour', *Journal of Substance Abuse Treatment*, 45: 155–62.

Decker, S. and Martino, S. (2013) 'Unintended effects on clinicians' interest, confidence and commitment in using MI', *Drug and Alcohol Dependence*, 132: 681–7.

Deighton, S. and Addington, J. (2013) 'Exercise practices in individuals at clinical high risk of developing psychosis', *Early Intervention in Psychiatry*, 9(4): 284–91.

Department of Health (2011) *A Report on Physical Activity for Health from the Four Home Countries' Chief Medical Officers*. Available at: www.gov.uk/government/publications/start-active-stay-active-a-report-on-physical-activity-from-the-four-home-countries-chief-medical-officers (accessed 25 August 2016).

Department of Health (2014) *Closing the Gap: Priorities for Essential Change in Mental Health*. Available at: www.gov.uk/government/uploads/system/uploads/attachment_data/file/281250/Closing_the_gap_V2_-_17_Feb_2014.pdf (accessed 25 August 2016).

Di Forti, M., Morgan, C., Dazzan, P. et al. (2009) 'High-potency cannabis and the risk of psychosis', *The British Journal of Psychiatry*, 195(6): 488–91.

Di Forti, M., Sallis, H., Allegri, F. et al. (2014) 'Daily use, especially of high-potency cannabis, drives the earlier onset of psychosis in cannabis users', *Schizophrenia Bulletin*, 40(6): 1509–17.

Diabetes Prevention Program Research Group (2009) '10-year follow-up of diabetes incidence and weight loss in the Diabetes Prevention Program Outcomes Study', *The Lancet*, 374(9702): 1677–86.

Diabetes UK (2016) *What is Diabetes?* Available at: www.diabetes.org.uk/Guide-to-diabetes/What-is-diabetes/ (accessed 25 August 2016).

Dickens, G.L. and Stubbs, J.H. (2004) 'Smoking and mental health nurses: a survey of clinical staff in a psychiatric hospital', *Journal of Psychiatric and Mental Health Nursing*, 11: 445–51.

DiClemente, C.C., Schumann, K., Greene, P.A. and Earley, M.D. (2011) 'A transtheoretical model perspective on change: process-focussed intervention in mental health-substance use', in D. Cooper (ed.), *Mental Health-Substance Use: Intervention in Mental Health-Substance Use*. London: Radcliffe.

Dipasquale, S., Pariante, C.M., Dazzan, P. et al. (2013) 'The dietary pattern of patients with schizophrenia: a systematic review', *Journal of Psychiatric Research*, 47: 197–207.

Disability Rights Commission (2006) *Equal Treatment: Closing the Gap: A Formal Investigation into Physical Health Inequalities Experienced by People with Learning Disabilities and/or Mental Health Problems*. London: Disability Rights Commission. Available at: http://collections.europarchive.org/tna/20060924151545/drc-gb.org/newsroom/health_investigation.aspx (accessed 29 September 2016).

Dishman, R.K., Vandenberg, R.J., Motl, R.W. et al. (2009) 'Dose relations between goal setting, theory-based correlates of goal setting and increases in physical activity during a workplace trial', *Health Education Research*, doi:10.1093/her/cyp042.

Doherty, K. (2006) 'Giving up the habit', *Mental Health Today*, 6: 27–9.

Doll, R., Peto, R., Boreham, J. and Sutherland, I. (2004) 'Mortality in relation to smoking: 50 years' observations on male British doctors', *BMJ*, doi: 10.1136/bmj.38142.554479.AE.

Dragt, S., Nieman, D.H., Schultze-Lutter, F. et al. (2012) 'Cannabis use and age at onset of symptoms in subjects at clinical high risk for psychosis', *Acta Psychiatrica Scandinavica*, 125(1): 45–53.

Drake, R.E., Mueser, K.T. and Brunette, M.F. (2007) 'Management of persons with co-occurring severe mental illness and substance use disorder: programme implications', *World Psychiatry*, 6(3): 131–6.

Druss, B.G., Rosenheck, R.A., Desai, M.M. and Perlin, J.B. (2002) 'Quality of preventive medical care for patients with mental disorders', *Med. Care*, 40: 129–36.

Dube, S.R., Felitti, V.J., Dong, M. et al. (2003) 'Childhood abuse, neglect, and household dysfunction and the risk of illicit drug use: the adverse childhood experiences study', *Pediatrics*, 111(3): 564–72.

Dunlay, S.M., Thomas, R.J., Killian, J.M. and Roger, V.L. (2014) 'Participation in cardiac rehabilitation, readmissions, and death after acute myocardial infarction', *American Journal of Medicine*, 127(6): 538–46.

Dwyer, T., Bradshaw, J. and Happell, B. (2009) 'Comparison of mental health nurses' attitudes towards smoking and smoking behaviour', *International Journal of Mental Health Nursing*, 18: 424–33, and doi: 10.1111/j.1447-0349.2009.00628.x.

Ekelund, U., Ward, H.A., Norat, T. et al. (2015) 'Physical activity and all-cause mortality across levels of overall and abdominal adiposity in European men and women: the European Prospective Investigation into Cancer and Nutrition Study (EPIC)', *American Journal of Clinical Nutrition*, 101: 613–21.

Ekers, D., Richards, D. and Gilbody, S. (2008) 'A meta-analysis of randomized trials of behavioural treatment of depression', *Psychological Medicine*, 38(05): 611–23.

Esen-Danacı, A., Sarandöl, A., Taneli, F. et al. (2008) 'Effects of second generation antipsychotics on leptin and ghrelin', *Progress in Neuro-Psychopharmacology and Biological Psychiatry*, 32: 1434–8.

Faulkner, G., Taylor, A., Munro, S. et al. (2007) 'The acceptability of physical activity programming within a smoking cessation service for individuals with severe mental illness', *Patient Education and Counseling*, 66: 123–6.

Fergusson, D.M., Poulton, R., Smith, P.F. and Boden, J.M. (2006) 'Cannabis and psychosis', *BMJ*, 332: 172–5.

Fernandez-San-Martin, M.I., Martin-Lopez, L.M., Massa-Font, R. et al. (2014) 'The effectiveness of lifestyle interventions to reduce cardiovascular risk in patients with severe mental disorders: meta-analysis of intervention studies', *Community Ment. Health J.*, 50(1): 81–95.

Festiner, L. (1957) *A Theory of Cognitive Dissonance*. Stanford, CA: Stanford University Press.

Fidler, J.A. and West, R. (2009) 'Self-perceived smoking motives and their correlates in a general population sample', *Nicotine & Tobacco Research*, 11: 1182–8.

Fiedorowicz, G., Miller, J.D., Bishop, D.R. et al. (2012) 'Systematic review and meta-analysis of pharmacological interventions for weight gain from antipsychotics and mood stabilizers', *Curr. Psychiatry Rev.*, 8(1): 25–36.

Firth, J., Carney, R., Elliott, R. et al. (2016a) 'Exercise as an intervention for first-episode psychosis: a feasibility study', *Early Intervention in Psychiatry*. Available at: http://onlinelibrary.wiley.com/doi/10.1111/eip.12329/epdf (accessed 5 August 2016).

Firth, J., Carney, R., Jerome, L. et al. (2016b) 'The effects and determinants of exercise participation in first-episode psychosis: a qualitative study', *BMC Psychiatry*, 16: 1.

Firth, J., Rosenbaum, S., Stubbs, B. et al. (2016c) 'Motivating factors and barriers towards exercise in serious mental illness: a systematic review and meta-analysis', *Psychological Medicine*, 1: 1–13.

Firth, J., Rosenbaum, S., Stubbs, B. et al. (2016d) 'Preferences and motivations for exercise in early psychosis', *Acta Psychiatrica Scandinavica*, doi: 10.1111/acps.12562.

Firth, J., Cotter, J., Elliot, R. et al. (2015) 'A systematic review and meta-analysis of exercise interventions in schizophrenia patients', *Psychological Medicine*, 45(7): 1343–61.

Fleischhacker, W.W., Siu, C.O., Boden, R. et al. and EUFEST Study Group (2013) 'Metabolic risk factors in first-episode schizophrenia: baseline prevalence and course analysed from the European First-Episode Schizophrenia Trial', *International Journal of Neuropsychopharmacology*, 16: 987–95.

Foley, D. and Morley, K.I. (2011) 'Systematic review of early cardio-metabolic outcomes of the first treated episode of psychosis', *Archives of General Psychiatry*, 68(6): 609–16.

Fusar-Poli, P., Borgwardt, S., Bechdolf, A. et al. (2013) 'The psychosis high-risk state: a comprehensive state-of-the-art review', *JAMA Psychiatry*, 70(1): 107–20.

Fusar-Poli, P., Cappucciati, M., Rutigliano, G. et al. (2015a) 'At risk or not at risk? A meta-analysis of the prognostic accuracy of psychometric interviews for psychosis prediction', *World Psychiatry*, 14(3): 322–32.

Fusar-Poli, P., Díaz-Caneja, C., Patel, R. et al. (2015b) 'Services for people at high risk improve outcomes in patients with first episode psychosis', *Acta Psychiatrica Scandinavica*,133(1): 76–85.

Galletly, C.A., Foley, D.L., Waterreus, A. et al. (2012) 'Cardiometabolic risk factors in people with psychotic disorders: the second Australian national survey of psychosis', *Aust. N. Z. J. Psychiatry*, 46: 753–61.

Galling, B., Roldán, A., Nielsen, R.E. et al. (2016) 'Type 2 diabetes mellitus in youth exposed to antipsychotics: a systematic review and meta-analysis', *JAMA Psychiatry*, 73(3): 247–59.

Gangwisch, J.E., Malaspina, D., Albala, B.B. and Heymsfield, S.B. (2005) 'Inadequate sleep as a risk factor for obesity: analyses of the NHANES I', *Sleep*, 28(10): 1289–96.

Garber, A.J. (2012) 'Obesity and type 2 diabetes: which patients are at risk?', *Diabetes Obes. Metab.*, 14(5): 399–408.

Gates, J., Killackey, E., Phillips, L. and Álvarez-Jiménez, M. (2015) 'Mental health starts with physical health: current status and future directions of non-pharmacological interventions to improve physical health in first-episode psychosis', *The Lancet Psychiatry*, 2: 726–42.

Gilbody, S., Peckham, E., Man, M.-S. et al. (2015) 'Smoking cessation for people with severe mental ill health (SCIMITAR): results from a pilot randomised controlled trial', *The Lancet Psychiatry*, 2: 395–402.

Gill, K.E., Poe, L., Azimov, N. et al. (2013) 'Reasons for cannabis use among youths at ultra-high risk for psychosis', *Early Intervention in Psychiatry*, 9(3): 207–10.

Goldberg, R.W., Himelhoch, S., Kreyenbuhl, J. et al. (2005) 'Predictors of HIV and hepatitis testing and related service utilization among individuals with serious mental illness', *Psychosomatics*, 46: 573–7.

Goldstein, D.J. (1992) 'Beneficial health effects of modest weight loss', *Int. J. Obes. Relat. Metab. Disord.*, 16(6): 397–415.

Goodwin, P.J. and Stambolic, V. (2015) 'Impact of the obesity epidemic on cancer', *Ann. Rev. Med.*, 66: 281–96, and doi: 10.1146/annurev-med-051613-012328. Epub 12 November 2014.

Government Office for Science (2012) *Reducing Obesity: Future Choices – Mid-Term Review*. Available at: www.gov.uk/government/uploads/system/uploads/attachment_data/file/288025/12-1210-tackling-obesities-mid-term-review.pdf (accessed 25 August 2016).

Graeber, D.A., Moyers, T.B. and Griffith, G. (2003) 'A pilot study comparing motivational interviewing and an educational package in patients with schizophrenia and alcohol use disorders', *Community Mental Health Journal*, 36(3): 189–203.

Greaves, C.J., Sheppard, K.E., Abraham, C. et al. (2011) 'Systematic review of reviews of intervention components associated with increased effectiveness in dietary and physical activity interventions', *BMC Public Health*, 11: 119, and doi: 10.1186/1471-2458-11-119.

Greenwood, P. and Shiers, D. (2016) 'Don't just screen, intervene: a quality improvement initiative to improve physical health screening of young people experiencing severe mental illness in North West England', *Mental Health Review Journal*, 21: 1–13.

Guh, D.P., Zhang, W., Bansback, N. et al. (2009) 'The incidence of co-morbidities related to obesity and overweight: a systematic review and meta-analysis', *BMC Public Health*, 9: 88 and doi: 10.1186/1471-2458-9-88.

Gurillo, P., Jauhar, S., Murray, R.M. and MacCabe, J.H. (2015) 'Does tobacco use cause psychosis? Systematic review and meta-analysis', *The Lancet Psychiatry*, 2(8): 718–25.

Guthrie, B. and Morales, D.R. (2014) 'What happens when pay for performance stops?', *BMJ*, 348: g1413, and doi: 10.1136/bmj.g1413 (accessed 25 August 2016).

Hamer, M., Batty, D., Seldenrijk, A. and Kivimaki, M. (2011) 'Antidepressant medication use and future risk of cardiovascular disease: the Scottish Health Survey', *European Heart Journal*, 32: 437–42.

Hanson, M.D. and Chen, E. (2007) 'Socioeconomic status and health behaviors in adolescence: a review of the literature', *Journal of Behavioral Medicine*, 30(3): 263–85.

Happell, B., Platania-Phung, C. and Scott, D. (2011) 'Placing physical activity in mental health care: a leadership role for mental health nurses', *International Journal of Mental Health Nursing*, 20(5): 310–18.

Hardy, S. and Gray, R. (2010) 'Adapting the severe mental illness physical Health Improvement Profile for use in primary care', *International Journal of Mental Health Nursing*, 19: 350–5.

Hardy, S., Hinks, P. and Gray, R. (2014) 'Does training practice nurses to carry out physical health checks for people with severe mental illness increase the level of screening for cardiovascular risk?', *Int. J. Soc. Psychiatry*, 60: 236–42.

Hardy, S., White, J. and Gray, R. (2015) *The Health Improvement Profile: A Manual to Promote Physical Wellbeing in People with Severe Mental Illness*. Keswick: M&K Publishing.

Haskell, W.L., Lee, I.M., Pate, R.R., et al. (2007) 'Physical activity and public health: updated recommendation for adults from the American College of Sports Medicine and the American Heart Association', *Circulation*, 116: 1081.

Health Education England (2015) '*Raising the Bar: Shape of Caring': Health Education England*. Available at: www.google.co.uk/webhp?sourceid=chrome-instant&ion=1&espv=2&ie=UTF-8#q=Raising+the+Bar%3A+Shape+of+Caring (accessed 25 August 2016).

Health Survey for England (2016) *Health, Social Care and Lifestyles*. Available at: http://digital.nhs.uk/healthsurveyengland (accessed 25 August 2016).

Hettema, J.E. and Kirsch, J.T. (2011) 'Motivational interviewing: mental health-substance use', in D. Cooper (ed.), *Mental Health-Substance Use: Intervention in Mental Health-Substance Use*. London: Radcliffe.

Hippisley-Cox, J., Parker, C., Coupland, C. and Vinogradova, Y. (2007) 'Inequalities in the primary care of patients with coronary heart disease and serious mental health problems: a cross-sectional study', *Heart*, 93: 1256–62.

Hippocrates (1955) 'Hippocratic Writings', *Encyclopedia Britannica*.

Hodgekins, J., French, P., Birchwood, M. et al. (2015) 'Comparing time use in individuals at different stages of psychosis and a non-clinical comparison group', *Schizophrenia Research*, 161(2–3): 188–93.

Holt, R.I. and Peveler, R.C. (2009) 'Obesity, serious mental illness and antipsychotic drugs', *Diabetes Obesity and Metabolism*, 11: 665–79.

Howard, B.T., Iles, T.L., Coles, J.A. et al. (2015) 'Reversible and irreversible damage of the myocardium: ischemia/reperfusion injury and cardioprotection', in P.A. Iaizzo (ed.), *Handbook of Cardiac Anatomy, Physiology, and Devices*, 3rd edn. Switzerland: Springer International.

Howard, L. and Gamble, C. (2011) 'Supporting mental health nurses to address the physical health needs of people with serious mental illness in acute inpatient care settings', *Journal of Psychiatric and Mental Health Nursing*, 18: 105–12.

Howard, L.M., Barley, E.A., Davies, E. et al. (2010) 'Cancer diagnosis in people with severe mental illness: practical and ethical issues', *Lancet Oncol.*, 11: 797–804.

Hsu, J.H., Chien, I.C., Lin, C.H. et al. (2011) 'Incidence of diabetes in patients with schizophrenia: a population-based study', *Can. J. Psychiatry*, 56(1): 19–26. Available at: www.nhsemployers.org/your-workforce/primary-care-contacts/general-medical-services/quality-and-outcomes-framework (accessed 25 August 2016).

Hsu, W.C., Araneta, M.R.G., Kanaya, A.M. et al. (2015) 'BMI cut points to identify at-risk Asian Americans for type 2 diabetes screening', *Diabetes Care*, 38(1): 150–8.

Huber, C.G., Smieskova, R., Schroeder, K. et al. (2014) 'Evidence for an agitated-aggressive syndrome predating the onset of psychosis', *Schizophrenia Research*, 157(1–3): 26–32.

Huxley, R.R. and Neil, H.A.W. (2003) 'The relationship between dietary flavanol intake and coronary heart disease mortality: a meta-analysis of prospective cohort studies', *European Journal of Clinical Nutrition*, 57: 904–8.

International Diabetes Federation (2006) The IDF consensus worldwide definition of the metabolic syndrome. Available at: www.idf.org/metabolic-syndrome (accessed 25 August 2016).

International Physical Health in Youth (iphYs) Working Group (2013) *Healthy Active Lives (HeAL) Consensus Statement 2013*. Available at: www.iphys.org.au/home (accessed 3 October 2016).

Jakupcak, M., Wagner, A., Paulson, A. et al. (2010) 'Behavioral activation as a primary care-based treatment for PTSD and depression among returning veterans', *Journal of Traumatic Stress*, 23(4): 491–5.

Jamal, M., Willem Van der Does, A.J. and Cuijpers, P. (2012) 'Association of smoking and nicotine dependence with severity and course of symptoms in patients with depressive or anxiety disorder', *Drug and Alcohol Dependence*, 126(1–2): 138–46.

Jefferies, S., Weatherall, M., Young, P. and Beasley, R. (2011) 'A systematic review of the accuracy of peripheral thermometry in estimating core temperatures among febrile critically ill patients', *Crit. Care Resusc.*, 13(3): 194–249.

Jochelson, K. and Majrowski, B. (2006) *Clearing the Air: Debating SmokeFree Policies in Psychiatric Units*. London: King's Fund. Available at: www.kingsfund.org.uk/sites/files/kf/field/field_publication_file/clearing-the-air-debating-smoke-free-policies-psychiatric-units-karen-jochelson-bill-majrowski-kings-fund-18-july-2006.pdf (accessed 25 August 2016).

Johnson, J.L., Malchy, L.A., Ratner, P.A. et al. (2009) 'Community mental healthcare providers' attitudes and practices related to smoking cessation interventions for people living with severe mental illness', *Patient Educ. Couns.*, 77, 2: 289–95.

Kahn, R.S., Fleischhacker, W.W., Boter, H. et al. and EUFEST Study Group (2008) 'Effectiveness of antipsychotic drugs in first-episode schizophrenia and schizophreniform disorder: an open randomised clinical trial', *The Lancet*, 371: 1085–97.

Kanter, J., Busch, A. and Rusch, L. (2009) *Behavioral Activation*. London: Routledge.

Kavanagh, D.J., Young, R., White, A. et al. (2004) 'A brief motivational intervention for substance misuse in recent-onset psychosis', *Drug and Alcohol Review*, 23: 151–5.

Kay, S., Opler, L. and LindenMayer, J. (1989) 'The Positive and Negative Syndrome Scale (PANSS): rationale and standardisation', *British Journal of Psychiatry*, 155(suppl. 7): 59–67.

Killackey, E.J., Jackson, H.J., Gleeson, J. et al. (2006) 'Exciting career opportunity beckons! Early intervention and vocational rehabilitation in first-episode psychosis: employing cautious optimism', *Aust. N. Z. J. Psychiatry*, 40: 951–62.

Kimhy, D., Vakhrusheva, J., Bartels, M.N. et al. (2014) 'Aerobic fitness and body mass index in individuals with schizophrenia: Implications for neurocognition and daily functioning', *Psychiatry Research*, 220: 784–91.

King, P., Peacock, I. and Donnelly, R. (1998) 'The UK Prospective Diabetes Study (UKPDS): clinical and therapeutic implications for type 2 diabetes', *Br. J. Clin. Pharmacol.*, 48: 643–8.

Kirkbride, J.B., Jones, P.B., Ullrich, S. and Coid, J.W. (2014) 'Social deprivation, inequality and the neighbourhood-level incidence of psychotic syndromes in East London', *Schizophrenia Bulletin*, 40: 169–80.

Kirkbride, J.B., Errazuriz, A., Croudace, T.J. et al. (2012) 'Incidence of schizophrenia and other psychoses in England, 1950–2009: a systematic review and meta-analyses', *PLOS ONE*, 7(3): e31660, and doi: 10.1371/journal.pone.0031660.

Kirkbride, J.B., Fearon, P., Morgan, C. et al. (2006) 'Heterogeneity in incidence rates of schizophrenia and other psychotic syndromes: findings from the 3-center AeSOP study', *Archives of General Psychiatry*, 63: 250–8.

Kirkbride, J.B., Morgan, C., Fearon, P. et al. (2007) 'Neighbourhood-level effects on psychoses: re-examining the role of context', *Psychological Medicine*, 37: 1413–25.

Kisely, S., Crowe, E. and Lawrence, D. (2013) 'Cancer-related mortality in people with mental illness', *JAMA Psychiatry*, 70(2): 209–17.

Kluge, M., Schuld, A., Himmerich, H. et al. (2007) 'Clozapine and olanzapine are associated with food craving and binge eating: results from a randomized double-blind study', *J. Clin. Psychopharmacol.*, 27: 662–6.

Knowles, S., Bradshaw, T., Peckham, E. and Gilbody, S. (2016) 'Making the journey with me: a qualitative study of experiences of a bespoke mental health smoking cessation intervention for service users with serious mental illness', *BMC Psychiatry*, 16: 193.

Koivukangas, J., Tammelin, T., Kaakinen, M. et al. (2010) 'Physical activity and fitness in adolescents at risk for psychosis within the Northern Finland 1986 birth cohort', *Schizophrenia Research*, 116(2–3): 152–8.

Kumari, V. and Postma, P. (2005) 'Nicotine use in schizophrenia: the self-medication hypotheses', *Neuroscience and Biobehavioral Reviews*, 29(6): 1021–34.

Kuna, S.T., Reboussin, D.M., Borradaile, K.E. et al. (2013) 'Long-term effect of weight loss on obstructive sleep apnea severity in obese patients with type 2 diabetes', *Sleep*, 36(5): 641–9.

Labad, J., Stojanovic-Perez, A., Montalvo, I. et al. (2015) 'Stress biomarkers as predictors of transition to psychosis in at-risk mental states: roles for cortisol, prolactin and albumin', *Journal of Psychiatric Research*, 60: 163–9.

Lawn, S.J. (2004) 'Systemic barriers to quitting smoking among institutionalised public mental health service populations: a comparison of two Australian sites', *Int. J. Soc. Psychiatry*, 50(3): 204–15.

Lawrence, W., Black, C., Tinati, T. et al. (2016) '"Making every contact count": evaluation of the impact of an intervention to train health and social care practitioners in skills to support health behaviour change', *Journal of Health Psychology*, 21(2): 138–51.

Lee, E.H., Hui, C.L., Chang, W. et al. (2013) 'Impact of physical activity on functioning of patients with first-episode psychosis: a 6-months prospective longitudinal study', *Schizophrenia Research*, 150: 538–41.

Lee, E., Hui, C.L.M., Lai, D.C. et al. (2012) 'Association of psychopathology and physical activity in people with first-episode psychosis', *Early Intervention in Psychiatry*, 6: 73.

Leffingwell, T.R., Neumann, C.A., Babitzke, A.C. and Leedy, M.J. (2007) 'Social psychology and motivational interviewing: a review of relevant principles and recommendations for research and practice', *Behavioural and Cognitive Psychotherapy*, 35: 31–45.

Lejuez, C., Hopko, D., Acierno, R. et al. (2011) 'Ten-year revision of the brief behavioural activation for depression: revised treatment manual', *Behavior Modification*, 35(2): 111–61.

Leonard, M., Graham, S. and Bonacum, D. (2004) 'The human factor: the critical importance of effective teamwork and communication in providing safe care', *Qual. Saf. Health Care*, 13(Suppl 1): i85–i90.

Lester, H., Tritter, J.Q. and Sorohan, H. (2005) 'Patients' and health professionals' views on primary care for people with serious mental illness: focus group study', *BMJ*, 330: 1122.

Lewinsohn, P.M. and Graf, M. (1973) 'Pleasant activities and depression', *Journal of Consulting and Clinical Psychology*, 41(2): 261.

Lindamer, L.A., McKibbin, C., Norman, G.J. et al. (2008) 'Assessment of physical activity in middle-aged and older adults with schizophrenia', *Schizophrenia Research*, 104: 294–301.

Lindström, J., Peltonen, M., Eriksson, J.G. et al. and for the Finnish Diabetes Prevention Study (2013) 'Improved lifestyle and decreased diabetes risk over 13 years: long-term follow-up of the randomised Finnish Diabetes Prevention Study (DPS)', *Diabetologia*, 56: 284–93.

Livermore, N., Sharpe, L. and McKenzie, D. (2010) 'Panic attacks and panic disorder in chronic obstructive pulmonary disease: a cognitive behavioral perspective', *Respiratory Medicine*, 104(9): 1246–53.

Lovell, K., Wearden, A., Bradshaw, T. et al. (2014) 'An exploratory randomized controlled study of a healthy living intervention in early intervention services for psychosis: the INTERvention to encourage ACTivity, improve diet, and reduce weight gain (INTERACT) study', *Journal of Clinical Psychiatry*, 75(5): 498–505.

Lundahl, B.W. and Burke, B.L. (2009) 'The effectiveness and applicability of motivational interviewing: a practice-friendly review of four meta-analyses', *Journal of Clinical Psychology*, 65(11): 1232–45.

Lundahl, B.W., Kunz, C., Brownell, C. et al. (2010) A Meta-Analysis of Motivational Interviewing Twenty-Five Years of Empirical Studies. Research on Social Work Practice OnlineFirst, published on January 11, 2010 as doi:10.1177/1049731509347850

Lundahl, B., Moleni, T., Burke, B.L. et al. (2013) 'Motivational Interviewing in medical care settings: a systematic review and meta-analysis of randomised controlled trials', *Patient Education and Counseling*, 93: 157–68.

Luppino, F.S., de Wit, L.M., Bouvy, P.F. et al. (2010) 'Overweight, obesity, and depression: a systematic review and meta-analysis of longitudinal studies', *Arch. Gen. Psychiatry*, 67(3): 220–9.

MacPherson, L., Tull, M.T., Matusiewicz, A.K. et al. (2010) 'Randomized controlled trial of behavioral activation smoking cessation treatment for smokers with elevated depressive symptoms', *Journal of Consulting and Clinical Psychology*, 78(1): 55–61.

Magkos, F., Fraterrigo, G., Yoshino, J. et al. (2016) 'Effects of moderate and subsequent progressive weight loss on metabolic function and adipose tissue biology in Humans with obesity', *Cell Metab.*, 23(4): 591–601.

Mairs, H. (2017, in print) *Revisiting Negative Symptoms: Working with Reduced Expression and Activity in Psychosis*. London: Palgrave Macmillan.

Mairs, H.J., Lovell, K. and Keeley, P. (2012) 'Carer and mental health professional views of a psychosocial treatment for negative symptoms: a qualitative study', 49 (10): 1191–9.

Mairs, H.J., Lovell, K., Campbell, M. and Keeley, P. (2011) 'Development and pilot investigation of a behavioral activation for negative symptoms', *Behavior Modification*, 35(5): 486–506.

Manu, P., Dima, L., Shulman, M. et al. (2015) 'Weight gain and obesity in schizophrenia: epidemiology, pathobiology, and management', *Acta Psychiatr. Scand.*, 132: 97–108.

Marieb, E.N. and Hoehn, K. (2016) *Human Anatomy and Physiology*, 10th edn. London: Pearson Education.

Marques, T.R., Smith, S., Bonaccorso, S. et al. (2012) 'Sexual dysfunction in people with prodromal or first-episode psychosis', *British Journal of Psychiatry*, 201: 131–6.

Martino, S., Carrol, K.M., Charla, N. and Rounsaville, B.J. (2006) 'A randomised controlled pilot study of motivational interviewing for patients with psychotic and drug use disorders', *Journal of Addiction*, 101: 1479–92.

Marwaha, S.J., Bebbington, P., Stafford, M. et al. (2007) 'Rates and correlates of employment in people with schizophrenia in the UK, France and Germany', *British Journal of Psychiatry*, 191: 30–7.

Maudsley, H. (1879) *The Pathology of Mind*, 3rd edn. London: Macmillan.

McCloughen, A. (2003) 'The association between schizophrenia and cigarette smoking: a review of the literature and implications for mental health nursing practice', *International Journal of Mental Health Nursing*, 12: 119–29.

McCloughen, A., Foster, K., Kerley, D. et al. (2016) 'Physical health and well-being: Experiences and perspectives of young adult mental health consumers', *International Journal of Mental Health Nursing*. Available at: www.ncbi.nlm.nih.gov/pubmed/26856981 (accessed 25 August 2016).

McGorry, P.D., Yung, A.R., Phillips, L.J. et al (2002) 'Randomized controlled trial of interventions designed to reduce the risk of progression to first-episode psychosis in a clinical sample with subthreshold symptoms', *Arch. Gen. Psychiatry*, 59(10): 921–8

McIntyre, R.S., McCann, S.M. and Kennedy, S.H. (2001) 'Antipsychotic metabolic effects: weight gain, diabetes mellitus, and lipid abnormalities', *Can. J. Psychiatry*, 46: 273–81.

McManus, S., Meltzer, H. and Campion, J. (2010) *Cigarette Smoking and Mental Health in England: Data from the Adult Psychiatric Morbidity Survey 2007*. London: National Centre for Social Research. Available at: www.natcen.ac.uk/media/21994/smoking-mental-health.pdf (accessed 25 August 2016).

McNally, L. and Ratschen, E. (2010) 'The delivery of stop smoking support to people with mental health conditions: a survey of NHS stop smoking services', *BMC Health Services Research*, 10: 179, and doi: 10.1186/1472-6963-10-179.

McPherson, K., Britton, A. and Causer, L. (2002) *Coronary Heart Disease: Estimating the Impact of Changes in Risk Factors*. London: Stationery Office National Heart Forum.

Michie, S., Churchill, S. and West, R. (2011a) 'Identifying evidence-based competences required to deliver behavioural support for smoking cessation', *Annals of Behavioral Medicine*, 41(1): 59–70.

Michie, S., Hyder, N., Walia, A. and West, R. (2011b) 'Development of a taxonomy of behaviour change techniques used in individual behavioural support for smoking cessation', *Addictive Behaviors*, 36: 315–19.

Miller, W.R. (1983) 'Motivational interviewing with problem drinkers', *Behavioural Psychotherapy*, 11: 147–72.

Miller, W.R. and Moyers, T.B. (2006) 'Eight stages in learning motivational interviewing', *Journal of Teaching in the Addictions*, 5(1): 3–17.

Miller, W.R. and Rollnick, S. (1991) *Motivational Interviewing: Preparing People to Change Behaviour*. New York: Guilford Press.

Miller, W.R. and Rollnick, S. (2002) *Motivational Interviewing: Preparing People for Change*, 2nd edn. New York: Guilford Press.

Miller, W.R. and Rollnick, S. (2009) 'Ten things that motivational interviewing is not', *Behavioural and Cognitive Psychotherapy*, 37: 129–40.

Miller, W.R. and Rose, G. (2015) 'Motivational interviewing and decisional balance: contrasting responses to client ambivalence', *Behavioural and Cognitive Psychotherapy*, 43: 129–41.

Miller, W.R., Villanueva, M., Tonigan, J.S. and Cuzmar, I. (2007) 'Are special treatments needed for special populations?', *Alcohol Treatment Quarterly*, 25: 63–78.

Mitchell, A.J. and Hardy, S.A. (2013) 'Screening for metabolic risk among patients with severe mental illness and diabetes: a national comparison', *Psychiatr. Serv.*, 64: 1060–3.

Mitchell, A.J. and Lawrence, D. (2011) 'Revascularisation and mortality rates following acute coronary syndromes in people with severe mental illness: comparative meta-analysis', *British Journal of Psychiatry*, 198: 434–41.

Mitchell, A.J., Malone, D. and Doebbeling, C.C. (2009) 'Quality of medical care for people with and without comorbid mental illness and substance misuse: systematic review of comparative studies', *British Journal of Psychiatry*, 194: 491–9.

Mitchell, A.J., Espirito, I., Pereira, S. et al. (2014) 'Breast cancer screening in women with mental illness: comparative meta-analysis of mammography uptake', *British Journal of Psychiatry*, 205: 428–35.

Mitchell, A.J., Vancampfort, D., De Herdt, A. et al. (2013a) 'Is the prevalence of metabolic syndrome and metabolic abnormalities increased in early schizophrenia? A comparative meta-analysis of first-episode, untreated and treated patients', *Schizophrenia Bulletin*, 39(2): 295–305.

Mitchell, A.J., Vancampfort, D., Sweers, K. et al. (2013b) 'Prevalence of metabolic syndrome and metabolic abnormalities in schizophrenia and related disorders: a systematic review and meta-analysis', *Schizophrenia Bulletin*, 39(2): 306–18.

Mittal, V.A., Gupta, T., Orr, J.M. et al. (2013) 'Physical activity level and medial temporal health in youth at ultra-high risk for psychosis', *Journal of Abnormal Psychology*, 122(4): 1101–10.

Morabia, A. and Zhang, F.F. (2004) 'History of medical screening: from concepts to action', *Postgrad. Med. J.*, 80: 463–9.

Morgan, A.J., Parker, A.G., Álvarez-Jiménez, M. and Jorm, A.F. (2013) 'Exercise and mental health: an Exercise and Sports Science Australia Commissioned Review', *Journal of Exercise Physiology Online*, 16(4): 64–70.

Morgan, V., McGrath, J., Jablensky, A. et al. (2014) 'Psychosis prevalence and physical, metabolic and cognitive co-morbidity: data from the second Australian national survey of psychosis', *Psychological Medicine*, 44: 2163–76.

Mossaheb, N., Papageorgiou, K., Schäfer, M.R. et al. (2015) 'Changes in triglyceride levels in ultra-high risk for psychosis individuals treated with omega-3 fatty acids', *Early Intervention in Psychiatry*. Available at: https://dx.doi.org/10.1111/eip.12275 (accessed 25 August 2016).

Muller, D.C., Murphy, N., Johansson, M. et al. (2016) 'Modifiable causes of premature death in middle-age in Western Europe: results from the EPIC cohort study', *BMC Medicine*, doi: 10.1186/s12916-016-0630-6 (accessed 25 August 2016).

Myles, N., Newall, H., Curtis, J. et al. (2012) 'Tobacco use before, at and after first-episode psychosis: a systematic meta-analysis', *Journal of Clinical Psychiatry*, 73: 468–75.

Nash, M. (2014) *Physical Health and Well-Being in Mental Health Nursing: Clinical Skills for Practice*. Maidenhead: Open University Press.

National Centre for Smoking Cessation and Training (2014) Standard Treatment Programme: A guide to providing behavioural support for smoking cessation. http://www.ncsct.co.uk/shopdisp_a-standard-treatment-programme-for-smoking-cessation.php (accessed 3 October 2016)

National Heart, Lung and Blood Institute (2016) *What is Coronary Heart Disease?* Available at: www.nhlbi.nih.gov/health/health-topics/topics/cad (accessed 25 August 2016).

National Institute for Health and Care Excellence (NICE) (2008) *Cardiovascular Disease: Identifying and Supporting People Most at Risk of Dying Early, (PH15)*. Available at: www.nice.org.uk/guidance/ph15 (accessed 25 August 2016).

NICE (2009) *Depression: The Treatment and Management of Depression in Adults (Update) CG90*. London: NICE. Available at: www.nice.org.uk/Guidance/cg90 (accessed 25 August 2016).

NICE (2010) *Depression in Adults: Recognition and Management*. Available at: www.nice.org.uk/guidance/cg90/resources/depression-in-adults-recognition-and-management-975742636741 (accessed 25 August 2016).

NICE (2013a) *Myocardial Infarction: Cardiac Rehabilitation and Prevention of Further Cardiovascular Disease*. Available at: www.nice.org.uk/guidance/cg172 (accessed 25 August 2016).

NICE (2013b) *Psychosis and Schizophrenia in Children and Young People: Recognition and Management*. Available at: www.nice.org.uk/guidance/cg155 (accessed 25 August 2016).

NICE (2013c) *Smoking: Acute, Maternity and Mental Health Services*. Public Health Guideline, 27 November. Available at: nice.org.uk/guidance/ph48 (accessed 25 August 2016).

NICE (2014a) *Psychosis and Schizophrenia in Adults: Treatment and Management*. Available at: www.nice.org.uk/Guidance/CG178 (accessed 25 August 2016).

NICE (2014b) *Encouraging People to Have NHS Health Checks and Supporting them to Reduce Risk Factors*. Available at: www.nice.org.uk/advice/lgb15/chapter/what-nice-says (accessed 25 August 2016).

NICE (2015) *Psychosis and Schizophrenia in Adults: Quality Standard (QS80)*. Available at: www.nice.org.uk/guidance/qs80 (accessed 25 August 2016).

National Institute for Health Research, Collaboration for Leadership in Applied Health Research and Care (CLAHRC) for Greater Manchester (2013) *Improving the Physical Health Care of People with Severe and Enduring Mental Illness Manchester Mental Health and Social Care Trust Pilot Project Evaluation Report*. Salford: Salford Royal NHS Foundation Trust. Available at: http://clahrc-gm.nihr.ac.uk/wp-content/uploads/Mental-and-physical-health-evaluation-report-November-2013.pdf (accessed 25 August 2016).

National Obesity Observatory (2012) *Adult Obesity and Socioeconomic Status*. Available at: www.google.co.uk/webhp?sourceid=chrome-instant&ion=1&espv=2&ie=UTF-8#q=Adult+Obesity+and+Socioeconomic+Status (accessed 25 August 2016).

National Patient Safety Agency (NPSA) (2007) *The Fifth Report from the Patient Safety Observatory. Safer Care for the Acutely Ill Patient: Learning from Serious Incidents.* London: NPSA.

Naylor, C., Parsonage, M., McDaid, D. et al. (2012) *Long-Term Conditions and Mental Health the Cost of Co-morbidities*. London: King's Fund and Centre for Mental Health. Available at: www.kingsfund.org.uk/sites/files/kf/field/field_publication_file/long-term-conditions-mental-health-cost-comorbidities-naylor-feb12.pdf (accessed 25 August 2016).

Nelson, B., Yuen, H.P., Wood, S.J. et al. (2013) 'Long-term follow-up of a group at ultra-high risk ('prodromal') for psychosis: the PACE 400 study', *JAMA Psychiatry*, 70(8): 793–802.

NHS Choices (2016a) *BMI Healthy Weight Calculator*. Available at: www.nhs.uk/Tools/Pages/Healthyweightcalculator.aspx (accessed 25 August 2016).

NHS Choices (2016b) *What is a Mediterranean Diet?* Available at: www.nhs.uk/Livewell/Goodfood/Pages/what-is-a-Mediterranean-diet.aspx (accessed 25 August 2016).

NHS Choices (2016) Making every contact count. Available at: http://www.makingeverycontactcount.co.uk/ (accessed 3 October 2016).

NHS digital (2016) *Quality and Outcomes Framework*. Available at: http://digital.nhs.uk/qof (accessed 25 August 2016).

NHS Employers (2016) *Quality and Outcomes Framework*. Available at: www.nhsemployers.org/your-workforce/primary-care-contacts/general-medical-services/quality-and-outcomes-framework (accessed 25 August 2016).

NHS England (2015a) *Achieving Better Access to Mental Health Services by 2020*. London. Available at: www.google.co.uk/webhp?sourceid=chrome-instant&ion=1&espv=2&ie=UTF-8#q=Achieving+Better+Access+to+Mental+Health+Services+by+2020 (accessed 25 August 2016).

NHS England (2015b) *Commissioning for Quality and Innovation Guidance for 2015–16*. London. Available at: www.google.co.uk/webhp?sourceid=chrome-instant&ion=1&espv=2&ie=UTF-8#q=Commissioning+for+Quality+and+Innovation+Guidance+for+2015-16 (accessed 25 August 2016).

NHS England (2016a) *Improving the Physical Health of People with Mental Health Problems: Actions for Mental Health Nurses*. Available at: www.gov.uk/government/uploads/system/uploads/attachment_data/file/532253/JRA_Physical_Health_revised.pdf (accessed 25 August 2016).

NHS England (2016b) *Improving the Physical Health of People with Serious Mental Illness a Practical Toolkit*. Available at: www.england.nhs.uk/mentalhealth/wp-content/uploads/sites/29/2016/05/serious-mental-hlth-toolkit-may16.pdf (accessed 25 August 2016).

Niblett, P. (2015) *Statistics on Smoking: England 2015*. Health and Social Care Information Centre. Available at: http://digital.nhs.uk/catalogue/pub17526/stat-smok-eng-2015-rep.pdf (accessed 25 August 2016).

Nouchi, R., Taki, Y., Takeuchi, H. et al. (2014) 'Four weeks of combination exercise training improved executive functions, episodic memory, and processing speed in healthy elderly people: evidence from a randomized controlled trial', *Age*, 36: 787–99.

Nursing and Midwifery Council (2010) Standards for Pre-registration nursing education. 16/09/2010 ed. London: Nursing and Midwifery Council. https://www.nmc.org.uk/standards/additional-standards/standards-for-pre-registration-nursing-education/ (accessed 3 October 2016)

Nyboe, L., Vestergaard, C.H., Moeller, M.K. et al. (2015) 'Metabolic syndrome and aerobic fitness in patients with first-episode schizophrenia, including a 1-year follow-up', *Schizophrenia Research*, 168: 381–7.

O'Donoghue, B., Yung, A.R., Wood, S. et al. (2015) 'Neighbourhood characteristics and the rate of identification of young people at ultra-high risk for psychosis', *Schizophrenia Research*, 169(1–3): 214–16.

Office of National Statistics (2016) *National Life Tables, United Kingdom: 2012–2014*. Available at: www.ons.gov.uk/peoplepopulationandcommunity/birthsdeathsandmarriages/lifeexpectancies/bulletins/nationallifetablesunitedkingdom/2015-09-23#life-expectancy-at-birth (accessed 25 August 2016).

Overbaugh, K.J. (2009) 'Acute coronary syndrome', *American Journal of Nursing*, 109(5): 42–52.

Owen, N., Healy, G.N., Matthews, C.E. et al. (2010) 'Too much sitting: the population-health science of sedentary behavior', *Exercise and Sport Sciences Reviews*, 38(3): 105.

Pagoto, S., Bodenlos, J.S., Schneider, K.L. et al. (2008) 'Initial investigation of behavioral activation therapy for co-morbid major depressive disorder and obesity', *Psychotherapy: Theory, Research, Practice, Training*, 45(3): 410.

Pagoto, S., Schneider, K.L., Whited, M.C. et al. (2013) 'Randomized controlled trial of behavioral treatment for comorbid obesity and depression in women: the Be Active Trial', *International Journal of Obesity*, 37(11): 1427–34.

Parker, C., McNeill, A. and Ratschen, E. (2012) 'Tailored tobacco dependence support for mental health patients: a model for inpatient and community services', *Addiction*, 107: 18–25.

Parliamentary Office of Science and Technology (2015) *Parity of Esteem for Mental Health*, Postnote No. 485, January.

Peckham, E., Bradshaw, T.J., Brabyn, S. et al. (2015) 'Exploring why people with SMI smoke and why they want to quit: baseline data from the SCIMITAR RCT', *Journal of Psychiatric Nursing*, doi: 10.1111/jpm.12241.

Phelan, M., Stradins, L., Amin, D. et al. (2004) 'The physical health check: a tool for mental health workers', *Journal of Mental Health*, 13: 277–85.

Phelan, S.M., Burgess, D.J., Yeazel, M.W. et al. (2015) 'Impact of weight bias and stigma on quality of care and outcomes for patients with obesity', *Obes. Rev.*, 16(4): 319–26.

Pischon, T., Boeing, H., Hoffmann, K. et al. (2008) 'General and abdominal adiposity and risk of death in Europe', *N. Engl. J. Med.*, 359(20): 2105–20.

Prabhat, J. (2009) 'Avoidable global cancer deaths and total deaths from smoking', *Nature Reviews Cancer*, 9: 655–64.

Praharaj, S.K., Kusum, A., Goyal, J.N. and Sinha, S.K. (2011) 'Metformin for olanzapine-induced weight gain: a systematic review and meta-analysis', *Br. J. Clin. Pharmacol.*, 71(3): 377–82.

Prochaska, J.O. and DiClemente, C.C. (1984) *The Transtheoretical Approach: Crossing the Traditional Boundaries of Therapy*. Homewood, IL: Dow Jones-Irwin.

Public Health England (2016) *Local Health*. Available at: www.localhealth.org.uk/#l=en;v=map4 (accessed 25 August 2016).

Ratschen, E., Britton, J., Doody, G.A. et al. (2009) 'Tobacco dependence, treatment and smoke-free policies: a survey of mental health professionals' knowledge and attitudes', *General Hospital Psychiatry*, 31: 576–82.

Rawlinson, C. and Bradshaw, T. (2014) 'Smoking cessation in individuals prescribed clozapine: implications for the role of mental health workers', *Mental Health Nursing*, 34(1): 12–15.

Rector, N. (2014) 'CBT for medication resistant psychosis targeting negative symptoms', in C. Steel (ed.), *CBT for Schizophrenia*. Chichester: John Wiley and Sons.

Resuscitation Council (UK) (2015) *Guidelines and Guidance: The ABCDE Approach*, website. Available at: www.resus.org.uk/resuscitation-guidelines/abcde-approach/ (accessed 25 August 2016).

Rhodes, S., Richards, D.A., Ekers, D. et al. (2014) 'Cost and outcome of behavioural activation versus cognitive behaviour therapy for depression (COBRA): study protocol for a randomised controlled trial', *Trials*, 15: 29.

Richard, A., Rohrmann, S., Vandeleur, C.L. et al. (2015) 'Associations between fruit and vegetable consumption and psychological distress: results from a population-based study', *BMC Psychiatry*, 15:21, doi: 10.1186/s12888-015-0597-4.

Richards, D. and Whyte, M. (2011) *National Programme Student Materials to Support the Delivery of Training for Psychological Wellbeing Practitioners Delivering Low Intensity Interventions* (3rd edn). Available at: https://cedar.exeter.ac.uk/media/universityofexeter/schoolofpsychology/cedar/documents/Reach_Out_3rd_edition.pdf (accessed 3 October 2016).

Robson, D., Haddad, M., Gray, R. and Gournay, K. (2013) 'Mental health nursing and physical health care: a cross-sectional study of nurses' attitudes, practice, and perceived training needs for the physical health care of people with severe mental illness', *Int. J. Ment. Health Nurs.*, 22: 409–17.

Rogers, C.R. (1951) *Client-Centered Therapy*. Boston, MA: Houghton Mifflin.

Rogers, C.R. (1959) 'A theory of therapy, personality and interpersonal relationships as developed in the client-centered framework', in S. Koch (ed.), *Psychology: The Study of a Science*, Vol. 3: *Formulations of the Person and Social Contexts*. New York: McGraw-Hill.

Rogers, C.R. (1961) *On Becoming a Person*. Boston, MA: Houghton Mifflin.

Roland, M. (2004) 'Linking physicians' pay to the quality of care: a major experiment in the United Kingdom', *N. Engl. J. Med.*, 351(14): 1448–54.

Rollnick, S., Mason, P. and Butler, C. (1999) *Health Behaviour Change: A Guide for Practitioners*. Edinburgh: Churchill Livingstone.

Rose, G. (1981) 'Strategy of prevention: lessons from cardiovascular disease', *BMJ Clin. Res. Ed.*, 282: 1847–51.

Rosenbaum, S., Tiedemann, A., Ward, P.B. et al. (2015) 'Physical activity interventions: an essential component in recovery from mental illness', *British Journal of Sports Medicine*, 49: 1544–5.

Royal College of Physicians (RCP) (2012) *National Early Warning Score (NEWS): Standardising the Assessment of Acute-Illness Severity in the NHS*, Report of a Working Party. London: RCP.

RCP (2013) *Smoking and Mental Health*. Available at: https://cdn.shopify.com/s/files/1/0924/4392/files/smoking_and_mental_health_-_full_report_web.pdf?7537870595093585378 (accessed 25 August 2016).

Royal College of Psychiatrists (2013) 'Whole-person care: from rhetoric to reality – achieving parity between mental and physical health', Occasional Paper No. 88. London: Royal College of Psychiatrists. Available at: www.rcpsych.ac.uk/files/pdfversion/OP88xx.pdf (accessed 25 August 2016).

Royal College of Psychiatrists (2014) *Report of the Second Round of the National Audit of Schizophrenia (NAS)*. London: Healthcare Quality Improvement Partnership. Available at: www.rcpsych.ac.uk/pdf/FINAL%20report%20for%20the%20second%20round%20of%20the%20National%20Audit%20of%20Schizophrenia%20-%208.10.14v2.pdf (accessed 25 August 2016).

Rucker, D., Padwal, R., Li, S.K. et al. (2007) 'Long-term pharmacotherapy for obesity and overweight: updated meta-analysis', *BMJ*, 335(7631): 1194–9.

Ryan, M.C., Collins, P. and Thakore, J.H. (2003) 'Impaired fasting glucose tolerance in first-episode, drug-naive patients with schizophrenia', *American Journal of Psychiatry*, 160: 284–9.

Saari, K.M., Lindeman, S.M., Viilo, K.M. et al. (2005) 'A 4-fold risk of metabolic syndrome in patients with schizophrenia: the Northern Finland 1966 birth cohort study', *Journal of Clinical Psychiatry*, 66: 559–63.

Sale, J., Gignac, M. and Hawker, G. (2008) 'The relationship between disease symptoms, life events, coping and treatment, and depression among older adults with osteoarthritis', *Journal of Rheumatology*, 35(2): 335–42.

Scheewe, T., Backx, F., Takken, T. et al. (2013) 'Exercise therapy improves mental and physical health in schizophrenia: a randomised controlled trial', *Acta Psychiatrica Scandinavica*, 127: 464–73.

Schizophrenia Commission (2012) *The Abandoned Illness: A Report from the Schizophrenia Commission*. London: Rethink Mental Illness. Available at: www.google.co.uk/webhp?sourceid=chrome-instant&ion=1&espv=2&ie=UTF-8#q=The+abandoned+illness%3A+a+report+from+the+Schizophrenia+Commission (accessed 25 August 2016).

Senn, T.E. and Carey, M.P. (2009) 'HIV testing among individuals with a severe mental illness: review, suggestions for research, and clinical implications', *Psychol. Med.*, 39: 355–63.

Shahab, L. (2013) *Quick Wins: The Short-Term Benefits of Stopping Smoking: Full Report*, National Centre for Smoking Cessation and Training (NCSCT). Available at: www.ncsct.co.uk/usr/pub/Quick%20_wins_full_report.pdf (accessed 25 August 2016).

Shahab, L. and West, R. (2012) 'Differences in happiness between smokers, ex-smokers and never smokers: cross-sectional findings from a national household survey', *Drug Alcohol Dependancy*, 1, 121(1–2): 38–44.

Shiers, D. and Curtis, J. (2014) 'Cardiometabolic health in young people with psychosis', *The Lancet Psychiatry,* 1(7): 492–4.

Shiers, D. and Smith, J. (2014) 'Early intervention and the power of social movements: UK development of early intervention in psychosis as a social movement and its implications for leadership' in *Early Intervention in Psychiatry*: *EI of Nearly Everything for Better Mental Health*. John Wiley, Chichester, pp. 337–357.

Shiers, D.E., Rafi, I., Cooper, S.J. et al.. (2014) *Positive Cardiometabolic Health Resource: An Intervention Framework for Patients with Psychosis and Schizophrenia*, updated edn of 2012. Royal College of Psychiatrists. Available at: www.rcpsych.ac.uk/quality/nationalclinicalaudits/schizophrenia/nationalschizophreniaaudit/nasresources.aspx (accessed 25 August 2016).

Shuel, F., White, J., Jones, M. and Gray, R. (2010) 'Using the serious mental illness health improvement profile (HIP) to identify physical problems in a cohort of community patients: a pragmatic case series evaluation', *International Journal of Nursing Studies*, 47: 136–45.

Simmons, J. and Griffiths, R. (2014) *CBT for Beginners: A Practical Guide for Beginners*. London: Sage.

Simon, G.E., Katon, W.J., Lin, E.H.B. et al. (2007) 'Cost-effectiveness of systematic depression treatment among people with diabetes mellitus', *Archives of General Psychiatry*, 64(1): 65–72.

Smith, D.J., Langan, J., McLean, G. et al. (2013a) 'Schizophrenia is associated with excess multiple physical-health comorbidities but low levels of recorded cardiovascular disease in primary care: cross-sectional study', *BMJ Open*, 3: e002808, and doi: 10.1136/bmjopen-2013-002808.

Smith, D.J., Martin, D., Mclean, G. et al. (2013b) 'Multimorbidity in bipolar disorder and undertreatment of cardiovascular disease: a cross sectional study', *BMC Med.*, 11: 263.

Smith, G.B., Prytherch, D.R., Meredith, P. et al. (2013c) 'The ability of the National Early Warning Score (NEWS) to discriminate patients at risk of early cardiac arrest, unanticipated intensive care unit admission, and death', *Resuscitation*, 84(4): 465–70, and doi: 10.1016/j.resuscitation.2012.12.016.

Smith, J. and members of the SHAPE team (2015) *Supporting Health and Promoting Exercise (SHAPE) Project for Young People with Psychosis*, Worcestershire Health and Care NHS Trust. Available at: www.hacw.nhs.uk/our-services/early-intervention-service/shape/ (accessed 25 August 2016).

Smokefree NHS (n.d.) *How Smoking Affects your Body*. www.nhs.uk/smokefree/why-quit/smoking-health-problems (accessed 25 August 2016).

Soundy, A., Wampers, M., Probst, M. et al. (2013) 'Physical activity and sedentary behaviour in outpatients with schizophrenia: a systematic review and meta-analysis', *International Journal of Therapy and Rehabilitation*, 20: 588–96.

Stafford, M.R., Jackson, H., Mayo-Wilson, E. et al. (2013) 'Early interventions to prevent psychosis: systematic review and meta-analysis', *BMJ*, 346: f185.

Staring, A.B.P., ter Huurne, M.-A.B. and van der Gaag, M. (2013) 'Cognitive behavioural therapy for negative symptoms (CBT-n) in psychotic disorders: a pilot study', *Journal of Behavior Therapy and Experimental Psychiatry*, 44(3): 300–6.

Stead, L.F., Koilpillai, P. and Lancaster, T. (2015) 'Additional behavioural support as an adjunct to pharmacotherapy for smoking cessation', *Cochrane Database of Systematic Reviews*, 10, Art. No. CD009670, and doi: 10.1002/14651858.CD009670.pub3 (accessed 25 August 2016).

Stead, L.F., Perera, R., Bullen, C. et al. (2012) 'Nicotine replacement therapy for smoking cessation', *Cochrane Database of Systematic Reviews*, 11, Art. No. CD000146, and doi: 10.1002/14651858.CD000146.pub4 (accessed 25 August 2016).

Steg, G., James, S.K., Atar, D. et al. (2012) 'ESC guidelines for the management of acute myocardial infarction in patients presenting with ST-segment elevation: the Task Force on the Management of ST-Segment Elevation Acute Myocardial Infarction of the European Society of Cardiology (ESC)', *European Heart Journal*, 33(20): 2569–619, doi: 10.1093/eurheartj/ehs215.

Steinberg, M.L., Zeidonis, D.M., Krejci, J.A. and Brandon, T.H. (2004) 'Motivational interviewing with personalised feedback: a brief intervention for motivating smokers with schizophrenia to seek treatment for tobacco dependence', *Journal of Consulting and Clinical Psychology*, 72(4): 723–8.

Strassnig, M., Brar, J.S. and Ganguli, R. (2012) 'Health-related quality of life, adiposity, and sedentary behavior in patients with early schizophrenia: preliminary study', *Diabetes, Metabolic Syndrome and Obesity: Targets and Therapy*, 5: 389–94.

Stubbs, B., Vancampfort, D., De Hert, M. and Mitchell, A.J. (2015) 'The prevalence and predictors of type two diabetes mellitus in people with schizophrenia: a systematic review and comparative meta-analysis', *Acta Psychiatr. Scand.*, 132: 144–57.

Stubbs, B., Williams, J., Gaughran, F. and Craig, T. (2016) 'How sedentary are people with psychosis? A systematic review and meta-analysis', *Schizophrenia Research*, Available at: http://dx.doi.org/10.1016/j.schres.2016.01.034 (accessed 25 August 2016).

Sumithran, P. and Proietto, J. (2013) 'The defence of body weight: a physiological basis for weight regain after weight loss', *Clin. Sci.* (Lond.), 124(4): 231–41.

Tarricone, I., Ferrari-Gozzi, B., Serretti, A. et al. (2010) 'Weight gain in antipsychotic-naive patients: a review and meta-analysis', *Psychological Medicine*, 40: 187–200.

Teff, K.L. and Kim, S.F. (2011) 'Atypical antipsychotics and the neural regulation of food intake and peripheral metabolism', *Physiol. Behav.*, 104(4): 590–8.

Teff, K.L., Rickels, M.R., Grudziak, J. et al. (2013) 'Antipsychotic-induced insulin resistance and postprandial hormonal dysregulation independent of weight gain or psychiatric disease', *Diabetes*, 62: 3232–40.

Thim, T., Krarup, N.H., Grove, E.L. et al. (2012) 'Initial assessment and treatment with the Airway, Breathing, Circulation, Disability, Exposure (ABCDE) approach', *International Journal of General Medicine*, 5: 117–21.

Thomas, J.G., Bond, D.S., Phelan, S. et al. (2014) 'Weight-loss maintenance for 10 years in the National Weight Control Registry', *Am. J. Prev. Med.*, 46(1): 17–23.

Thompson, P.D., Buchner, D., Piña, I.L. et al. (2003) 'Exercise and physical activity in the prevention and treatment of atherosclerotic cardiovascular disease: a statement from the Council on Clinical Cardiology (Subcommittee on Exercise, Rehabilitation, and Prevention) and the Council on Nutrition, Physical Activity, and Metabolism (Subcommittee on Physical Activity)', *Circulation*, 107: 3109–16.

Thongsai, S., Gray, R. and Bressington, D. (2016) 'The physical health of people with schizophrenia in Asia: Baseline findings from a physical health check programme', *J. Psychiatr. Ment. Health Nurs.*, Available at: www.ncbi.nlm.nih.gov/pubmed/27090192 (accessed 25 August 2016).

Thornicroft, G. (2011) 'Physical health disparities and mental illness: the scandal of premature mortality', *British Journal of Psychiatry*, 199: 441–2.

Thyer, B.A. and Irvine, S. (1984) 'Contingency management of exercise by chronic schizophrenic patients', *Perceptual and Motor Skills*, 58: 419–25.

Thygesen, K., Alpert, J.S. and White, H.D., on behalf of the Joint ESC/ACCF/AHA/WHF Task Force for the Redefinition of Myocardial Infarction (2007) 'Universal definition of myocardial infarction', *J. Am. Coll. Cardiol.*, 50(22): 2173–95.

Townsend, N., Bhatnagar, P., Wilkins, E. et al. (2015) *Cardiovascular Disease Statistics*, Britsh Heart Foundation. Available at: www.bhf.org.uk/publications/statistics/cvd-stats-2015 (accessed 25 August 2016).

Tsai, K.Y., Lee, C.C., Chou, Y.M. and Chou, F.H. (2012) 'Incidence and relative risk of stroke in patients with schizophrenia: a five-year follow-up study', *Schizophrenia Research* 138(1): 41–7.

Uttinger, M., Koranyi, S., Papmeyer, M. et al. (2014) 'Psychosis early detection: helpful or stigmatizing experience? A qualitative pilot study', *Schizophrenia Research*, 153: S270–1.

Vamos, E.P., Mucsi, I., Keszei, A. et al. (2009) 'Comorbid depression is associated with increased healthcare utilization and lost productivity in persons with diabetes: a large nationally representative Hungarian population survey', *Psychosomatic Medicine*, 71(5): 501–7.

van der Berg, J.D., Stehouwer, C.D., Bosma, H. et al. (2016) 'Associations of total amount and patterns of sedentary behavior with type 2 diabetes and the metabolic syndrome: the Maastricht Study', *Diabetologia*, online 2 February: 1–10 and doi: 10.1007/s00125-015-3861-8.

van der Gaag, M., Smit, F., Bechdolf, A. et al. (2013) 'Preventing a first episode of psychosis: meta-analysis of randomized controlled prevention trials of 12 month and longer-term follow-ups', *Schizophrenia Research*, 149(1–3): 56–62.

van Dijk, S.J., Tellam, R.L., Tellam, R.L. et al. (2015) 'Recent developments on the role of epigenetics in obesity and metabolic disease', *Clin. Epigenetics*, 7: 66.

Vancampfort, D., De Hert, M., Sweers, K. et al. (2013) 'Diabetes, physical activity participation and exercise capacity in patients with schizophrenia', *Psychiatry and Clinical Neurosciences*, 67: 451–6.

Vancampfort, D., Probst, M., Knapen, J. et al. (2012) 'Associations between sedentary behaviour and metabolic parameters in patients with schizophrenia', *Psychiatry Research*, 200: 73–8.

Vancampfort, D., Guelinckx, H., Probst, M. et al. (2015a) 'Aerobic capacity is associated with global functioning in people with schizophrenia', *Journal of Mental Health*, 24: 214–18.

Vancampfort, D., Rosenbaum, S., Probst, M. et al. (2015b) 'Promotion of cardiorespiratory fitness in schizophrenia: a clinical overview and meta-analysis', *Acta Psychiatrica Scandinavica*, 132: 131–43.

Vancampfort, D., Rosenbaum, S., Schuch, F.B. et al. (2015c) 'Prevalence and predictors of treatment dropout from physical activity interventions in schizophrenia: a meta-analysis', *General Hospital Psychiatry*, 39: 15–23.

Vancampfort, D., Stubbs, B., Mitchell, A.J. et al. (2015d) 'Risk of metabolic syndrome and its components in people with schizophrenia and related psychotic disorders, bipolar disorder and major depressive disorder: a systematic review and meta-analysis', *World Psychiatry*, 14: 339–47.

Vandenberghe, F., Gholam-Rezaee, M., Saiqi-Morqui, N. et al. (2015) 'Importance of early weight changes to predict long-term weight gain during psychotropic drug treatment', *Journal of Clinical Psychiatry*, 76: e1417-23, and doi: 10.4088/JCP.14m09358.

Varese, F., Smeets, F., Drukker, M. et al. (2012) 'Childhood adversities increase the risk of psychosis: a meta-analysis of patient-control, prospective-and cross-sectional cohort studies', *Schizophrenia Bulletin*, 38(4): 661–71.

Vincent, H.K., Heywood, K., Connelly, J. and Hurley, R.W. (2012) 'Obesity and weight loss in the treatment and prevention of osteoarthritis', *PMR*, 4(5): S59–67.

Waller, H., Garety, P., Jolley, S. et al. (2013) 'Low-intensity cognitive behavioural therapy for psychosis: a pilot study', *Journal of Behaviour Therapy and Experimental Psychiatry*, 44(1): 98–104.

Walther, S., Stegmayer, K., Horn, H. et al. (2014) 'Physical activity in schizophrenia is higher in the first episode than in subsequent ones', *Front Psychiatry*, 5: 3389.

Westbrook, D., Kennerley, H. and Kirk, J. (2011) *An Introduction to Cognitive Behavioural Therapy: Skills and Application*. London: Sage.

White, J. (2010) 'Evaluation of the serious mental illness Health Improvement Profile (HIP): the HIP 100', Paper presented at the 16th International Network for Psychiatric Nursing Research (NPNR) Conference: Collaborative Research and Partnership Working, 23 September, Oxford University.

White, J. (2015) 'Physical health checks in serious mental illness: a programme of research in secondary care', PhD thesis, University of East Anglia.

White, J., Gray, R. and Jones, M. (2009) 'The development of the serious mental illness physical Health Improvement Profile', *Journal of Psychiatric and Mental Health Nursing*, 16: 493–8.

White, J., Hemingway, S. and Stephenson, J. (2014) 'Training mental health nurses to assess the physical health needs of mental health service users: a pre- and post-test analysis', *Perspectives in Psychiatric Care*, 50: 243–50.

Whitlock, G., Lewington, S., Sherliker, P. et al. (2009) 'Body-mass index and cause-specific mortality in 900 000 adults: collaborative analyses of 57 prospective studies', *The Lancet*, 373(9669): 1083–96.

Williams, R.L., Wood, L.G., Collins, C.E. and Callister, R. (2015) 'Effectiveness of weight loss interventions – is there a difference between men and women: a systematic review', *Obes. Rev.*, 16(2): 171–86.

World Health Organization (WHO) (2007) *BMI Classification*. Available at: www.who.int/bmi/index.jsp?introPage=intro_3.html (accessed 25 August 2016).

WHO (2009) *Global Health Risks: Mortality and Burden of Disease Attributable to Selected Major Risks*. Available at: www.google.co.uk/webhp?sourceid=chrome-instant&ion=1&espv=2&ie=UTF-8#q=mortality%20and%20burden%20of%20disease%20attributable%20to%20selected%20major%20risks (accessed 25 August 2016).

WHO (2015) *World Health Statistics: Life Expectancy at Birth*. Available at: www.who.int/gho/en/ (accessed 25 August 2016).

WHO (2016a) *Global Report on Diabetes*. Available at: http://apps.who.int/iris/bitstream/10665/204871/1/9789241565257_eng.pdf?ua=1andua=1 (accessed 25 August 2016).

WHO (2016b) *Obesity and Overweight: Fact Sheet*. Updated June 2016. Available at: www.who.int/mediacentre/factsheets/fs311/en/ (accessed 25 August 2016).

WHO (2016c) *Tobacco Fact Sheet*. Updated June 2016. Available at: www.who.int/mediacentre/factsheets/fs339/en/ (accessed 25 August 2016).

Wu, Y., Zhai, L. and Zhang, D. (2014) 'Sleep duration and obesity among adults: a meta-analysis of prospective studies', *Sleep Med.* 15(12): 1456–62.

Yung, A.R. and McGorry, P.D. (1996) 'The prodromal phase of first-episode psychosis: past and current conceptualizations', *Schizophrenia Bulletin*, 22(2): 353–70.

Yung, A.R., Phillips, L.J., Yuen, H.P. et al. (2003) 'Psychosis prediction: 12-month follow up of a high-risk ('prodromal') group', *Schizophrenia Research*, 60(1): 21–32.

Yung, A.R., Phillips, L.J., Yuen, H.P. et al. (2004) 'Risk factors for psychosis in an ultra-high risk group: psychopathology and clinical features', *Schizophrenia Research*, 67(2): 131–42.

Yung, A.R., Yuen, H.P., McGorry, P.D. et al. (2005) 'Mapping the onset of psychosis: the comprehensive assessment of at-risk mental states', *Aust. N. Z. J. Psychiatry*, 39(11–12): 964–71.

Zhang, J.-P. and Malhotra, A.K. (2011) 'Pharmacogenetics and antipsychotics: therapeutic efficacy and side effects prediction – expert opinion', *Drug Metabolism and Toxicology*, 7: 9–37.

# INDEX

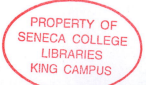